COOKBOOK

Mediterranean diet

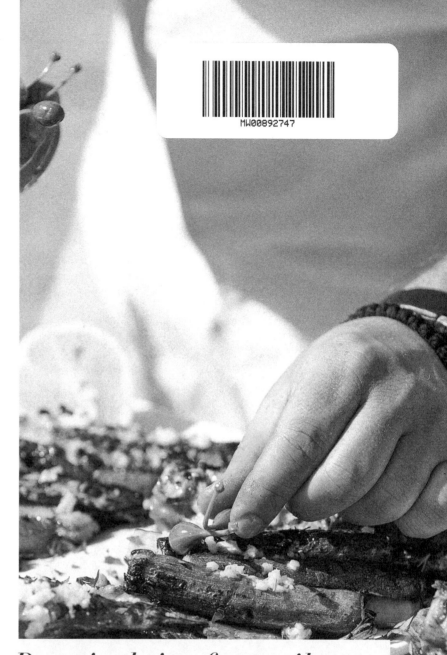

Practical tips for easily integrating the Mediterranean diet into your daily life, with lots of tasty and healthy kitchen-tested recipes.

RACHEL RODRIGUEZ

SCROLL TO THE END AND SCAN THE QR CODE TO ACCESS YOUR BONUSES

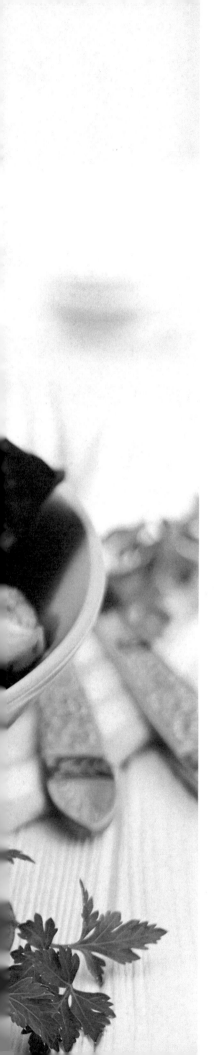

Table *of* CONTENT

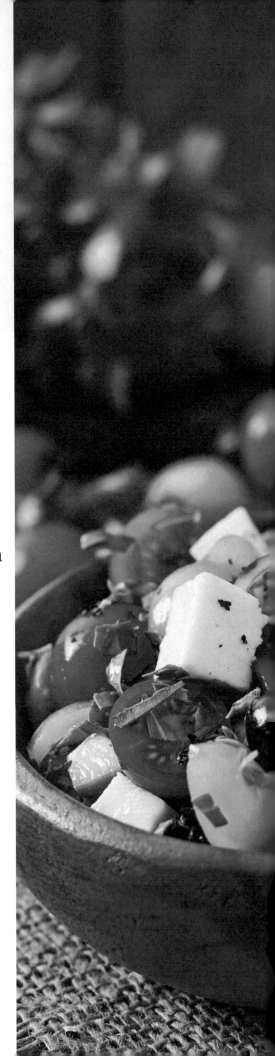

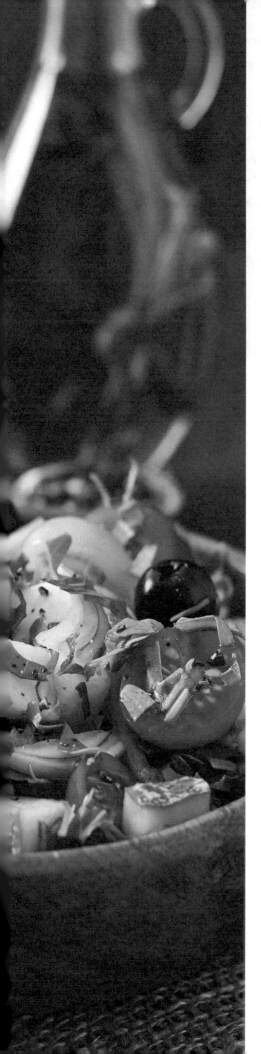

Table of CONTENT

WELCOME TO THIS JOURNEY OF HEALTH AND WELLNESS

Rachel Rodriguez

20+ years of experience

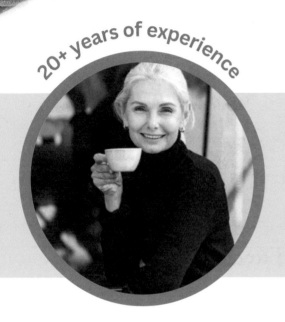

My name is Rachel Rodriguez. I am a dietitian and author. I welcome you on the journey to discover the Mediterranean diet, not just as a dietary regimen but as a valid lifestyle that celebrates abundant natural flavors and the joy of sharing food.

This book is an invitation to explore the Mediterranean diet not merely as a recommended list of foods but as an opportunity to rediscover the pleasure of eating well and with enthusiasm. I will introduce you to the fundamental principles of this diet, the foods to favor and those to limit, offering you a glimpse into the Mediterranean food pyramid. This model has stood the test of time and continues to be praised for its invaluable health benefits.

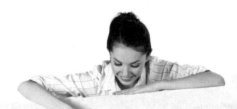

Immerse yourself with me in this journey, where food becomes an expression of Health and happiness, and let the Mediterranean diet inspire you to transform the way you think about, prepare, and savor food.

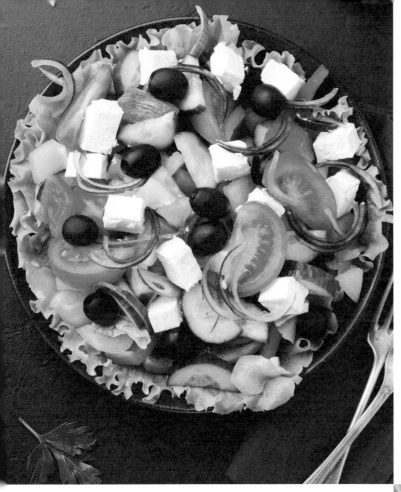

THE BENEFITS OF THE MEDITERRANEAN DIET AND THE REGIONS INVOLVED

The Mediterranean diet transcends a mere checklist of consumable items; it embodies a historical tradition that mirrors the culinary practices across various regions bordering the Mediterranean Sea. This nutritional blueprint is deeply rooted in the gastronomic customs of countries like Italy, Greece, Spain, and Portugal, as well as the southern parts of France, sections of the Middle East, and North Africa - notably Morocco, Algeria, Tunisia, and Lebanon. Each region injects its distinctive blend of flavors and ingredients, sharing core principles prioritizing fresh, minimally processed, and locally sourced foods.

UNESCO has recognized the Mediterranean diet as an Intangible Cultural Heritage of Humanity. This diet celebrates a way of life that harmonizes the bounty of the land with the rhythms of the seasons and the joys of shared meals. This accolade underscores the diet's significance as a means to physical wellness and sustainable cultural practice that nurtures community and environmental stewardship.

- **Health Benefits:** Research validates the myriad health benefits attributed to this diet, including:
- **Longevity:** The generous intake of fruits, vegetables, and healthy fats correlates with increased life expectancy and diminished prevalence of chronic diseases.
- **Heart Health:** A diet rich in monounsaturated fatty acids, mainly from olive oil, along with omega-3 fatty acids primarily sourced from fish, supports a robust cardiovascular system.
- **Weight Management:** This dietary approach fosters healthy weight management without the need for severe calorie restriction by emphasizing nutrient-dense and fulfilling foods.

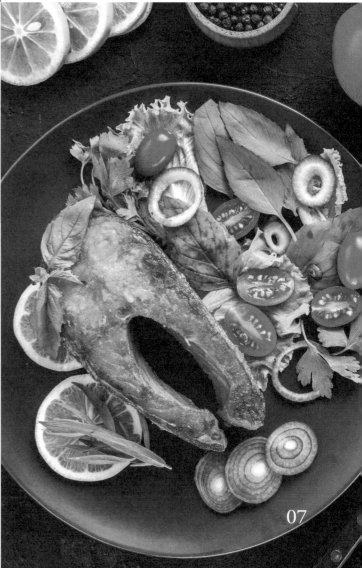

- **Diabetes Prevention:** The incorporation of whole grains and legumes, abundant in fiber, alongside a moderated sugar intake, aids in stabilizing blood glucose levels.
- **Mental Health:** Some studies have drawn connections between the Mediterranean diet and lower instances of depression and cognitive decline.

The recipes curated in this book are deeply ingrained in this venerable tradition, establishing a direct correlation between the earth's vitality and the individual's wellness. Each culinary encounter is a homage to fresh, seasonal produce, mirroring the age-old cycles that have steered the Mediterranean diet through the centuries.

This book serves as your passport to a dietary philosophy that is nurturing for the body and soothing for the soul. It features dishes that foster health and connect you to a rich tapestry of cultural heritage. Together, we will unveil how health can be infused into every morsel and how the culinary traditions of the Mediterranean can embellish our tables and our lives. The recipes detailed herein are tailored for seamless integration into daily routines, enabling you to reap the diet's benefits without preceding the delights and communal joy of eating. As we turn these pages, we celebrate the diversity of foods, mastering the art of crafting balanced meals that pay homage to the enduring principles of this UNESCO-recognized diet.

The Structure of the Mediterranean Diet - The Food Pyramid

At the heart of the Mediterranean diet lies its food pyramid, a nutritional model designed to guide us through daily choices and teach us the frequency and quantity in which to consume each type of food.

The base of the pyramid: this fundamental section recommends consuming various nutrient-rich plant foods daily.

- **Vegetables and Fruits:** To be enjoyed abundantly at every meal, they are a vital source of vitamins, minerals, fiber, and phytonutrients.

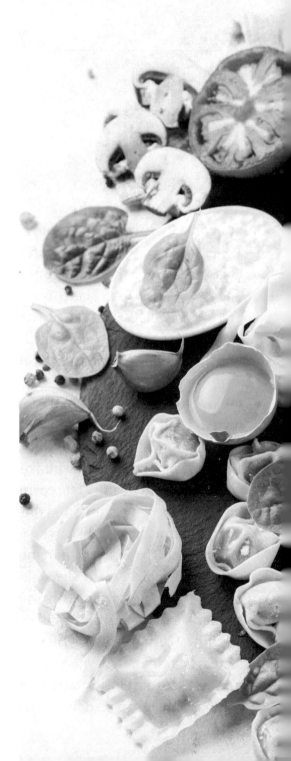

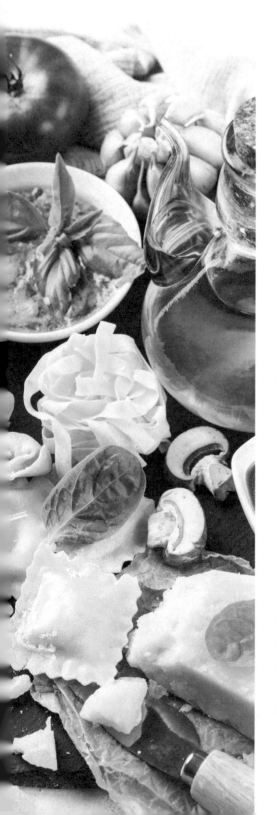

- **Whole Grains:** Whole-grain bread, pasta, rice, and cereals like barley and quinoa provide sustained energy and promote proper fiber intake.

- **Legumes, Nuts, and Seeds:** Beans, lentils, chickpeas, nuts, almonds, and seeds are rich in plant proteins, healthy fats, and other essential nutrients.

- **Olive Oil is the beating heart of the diet.** It is the main source of fats and is recommended to be used daily in place of other fats.

The central section of the pyramid focuses on foods to be consumed in moderate quantities, ideal for weekly consumption.

- **Fish and Seafood:** Suggested at least twice a week, they are rich in omega-3 fatty acids.

- **Dairy Products:** Cheese and yogurt, preferably low-fat, should be consumed in moderation, from daily to weekly.

- **Eggs and Poultry** are considered alternative protein sources. Moderate portions a few times a week are recommended.

The tip of The pyramid: At the apex, those foods are savored sparingly.

- **Red Meats:** Red meat should be consumed only occasionally and in small quantities.

- **Sweets and Added Sugars:** Sweets and foods with added sugars are considered occasional treats reserved for celebrations.

- **Wine:** Although wine can have a place in the Mediterranean diet, its consumption should be limited and consistently associated with meals.

Non-food elements: The Mediterranean diet also includes lifestyle aspects that go beyond food. It emphasizes the importance of regular physical activity and sharing meals with friends and family, promoting a holistic approach to well-being.

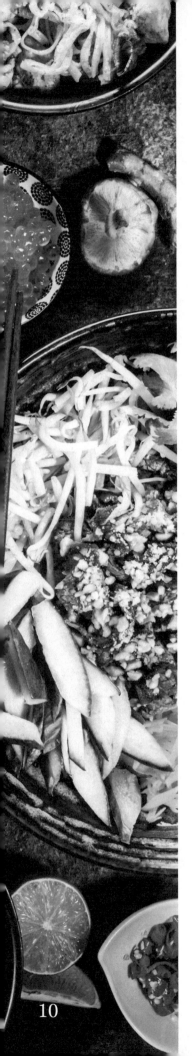
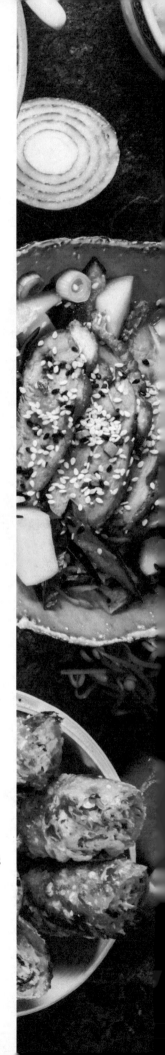

Mediterranean Recipes - Tradition and Health on the Plate

Welcome to the vibrant core of our culinary journey: the recipes. This chapter is a tribute to the diversity and abundance of the Mediterranean diet, a bridge linking the ancient wisdom of our lands to our modern lifestyle. Through the recipes we present, you'll discover how each ingredient is chosen for its nutritional profile and ability to transform a simple meal into a whole sensory experience. The dishes we explore are more than just culinary instructions; they are stories told through flavors, colors, and scents.

You will be guided step by step in preparing dishes that make the Mediterranean diet one of the healthiest and most delightful in the world.

These pages celebrate the most genuine ingredients and the most harmonious combinations, inspired by tradition yet adapted to fit the rhythm of modern life. Each recipe is designed to be accessible, whether you are an experienced cook or a novice at the stove, with variations and tips to make each dish suitable for your personal needs, never losing sight of the nutritional balance that is the hallmark of the Mediterranean diet.

These recipes are meant to nourish the body and the spirit, inviting you to rediscover the joy of home cooking and the value of sharing food with friends and family. The art of Mediterranean cooking is also an act of community and sharing, where the meal becomes a moment of union and exchange.

So, I invite you to read, cook, and experiment, making these recipes a window to Health and the joy of living. Let's open this culinary chapter together and be inspired by the world's most beloved diet.

Bon voyage and bon appétit!

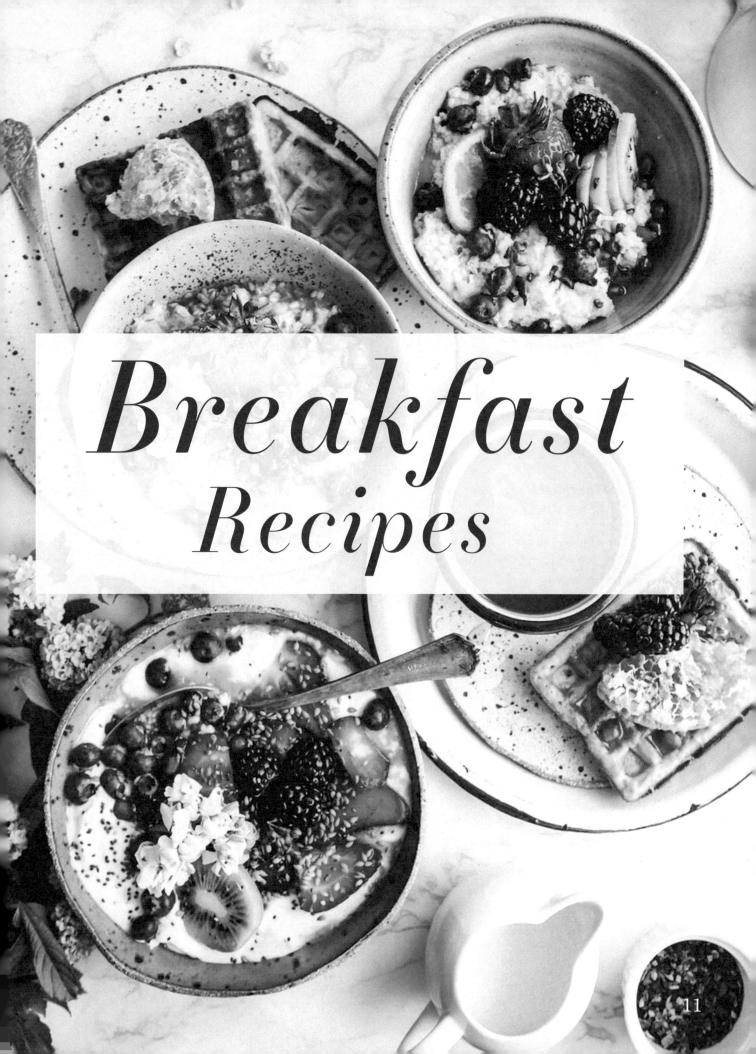

Breakfast
Recipes

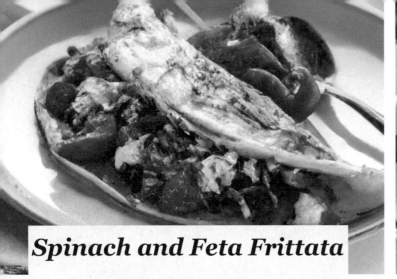

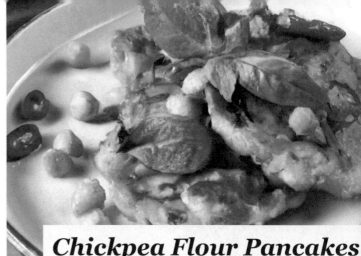

Spinach and Feta Frittata

Chickpea Flour Pancakes with Vegetables

(Greece)

(Italy)

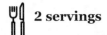 2 servings   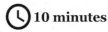 10 minutes   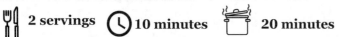 20 minutes

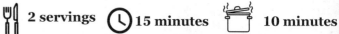 2 servings   15 minutes   10 minutes

INGREDIENTS

- 4 large eggs
- 1/2 cup milk
- 1/2 cup crumbled feta cheese
- 1 cup chopped fresh spinach
- 1/2 cup cherry tomatoes, halved
- 1 small red onion, thinly sliced
- 2 tablespoons extra virgin olive oil
- Salt and black pepper, to taste

INGREDIENTS

- 1 cup chickpea flour
- 1 1/4 cups water
- 1 small zucchini, grated
- 1/2 red bell pepper, diced
- 2 tablespoons red onion, finely chopped
- 1/4 teaspoon salt
- 1/4 teaspoon black pepper
- Olive oil for cooking

DIRECTIONS

Start by whisking the eggs with the milk, adding a pinch of salt and pepper to season until you achieve a smooth and uniform mixture. Heat the olive oil in a medium non-stick skillet over medium heat and add the finely sliced red onion, sautéing gently until it becomes soft and translucent. Then add the spinach, cooking it just enough to wilt it, before evenly distributing the cherry tomatoes and crumbled feta over the surface. Gently pour the egg mixture into the skillet, ensuring it covers the vegetables and feta evenly. Cook without stirring for about 5 minutes, then cover the skillet and reduce the heat, continuing to cook for another 10-15 minutes until the frittata is set and golden. Serve the frittata warm in the skillet for a flavorful and hearty start to the day.

DIRECTIONS

Mix the chickpea flour with water in a bowl until you get a smooth batter. Stir in the grated and chopped vegetables - zucchini, red bell pepper, and red onion - and season with salt and pepper. Heat a non-stick pan over medium heat and lightly grease it with olive oil. Pour a portion of the batter into the hot pan, forming pancakes about 4 inches in diameter. Cook for 4-5 minutes on each side until golden and crispy at the edges. Repeat with the remaining batter, adding more oil to the pan if necessary. Serve the pancakes warm, accompanied by a sauce or dressing of your choice.

CALORIES 320 KCAL	PROTEIN 18G	FATS 24G	FIBRE 2G

CALORIES 290 KCAL	PROTEIN 13G	FATS 6G	FIBRE 8G

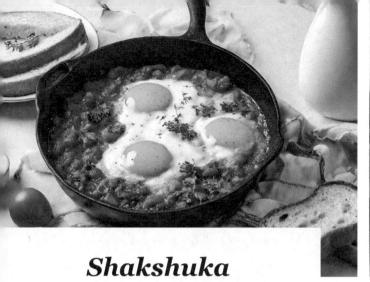

Shakshuka

(Morocco)

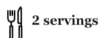 2 servings 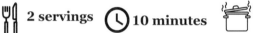 10 minutes 25 minutes

INGREDIENTS

- 4 large eggs
- 1 can (14 oz) peeled tomatoes
- 1 medium onion, thinly sliced
- 1 red bell pepper, cut into strips
- 2 cloves garlic, minced
- 2 tablespoons tomato paste
- 1 teaspoon ground cumin
- 1 teaspoon sweet paprika
- 1/2 teaspoon chili powder (optional)
- Salt and black pepper, to taste
- 3 tablespoons olive oil
- Fresh parsley or cilantro for garnish

DIRECTIONS

In a large skillet, heat the olive oil over medium heat. Add the onion and bell pepper, cooking until they soften, about 5-7 minutes. Incorporate the garlic, tomato paste, cumin, paprika, and chili powder, cooking for another 2 minutes until the spices are fragrant. Pour the peeled tomatoes, lightly crushing them with a spoon, and season with salt and pepper. Simmer the sauce on low heat for 10-15 minutes until it thickens slightly. Make small wells in the sauce with a spoon and crack an egg into each. Cover the skillet and cook until the eggs are done to your liking, for about 6-8 minutes, for soft eggs. Garnish with chopped fresh parsley or cilantro before serving.

CALORIES 250 KCAL	PROTEIN 12 G	FATS 14 G	FIBRE 4 G

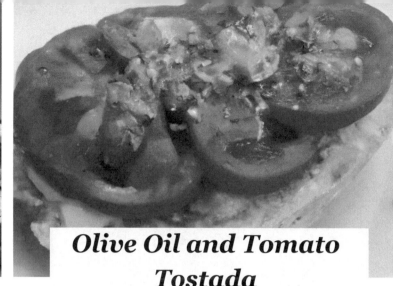

Olive Oil and Tomato Tostada

(Spain)

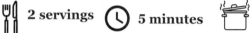 2 servings 5 minutes 5 minutes

INGREDIENTS

- 4 slices of whole wheat bread
- 2 ripe tomatoes, grated
- 2 tablespoons extra virgin olive oil
- Salt, to taste
- 1 clove of garlic (optional)

DIRECTIONS

Toast the bread slices until crispy and golden. If desired, lightly rub a garlic clove on one side of each toasted bread slice for extra flavor. Evenly distribute the grated tomatoes over the bread slices, covering the surface well. Season with a pinch of salt and a generous extra virgin olive oil drizzle. Serve immediately to enjoy their crunchiness.

CALORIES 200KCAL	PROTEIN 6G	FATS 7G	FIBRE 5G

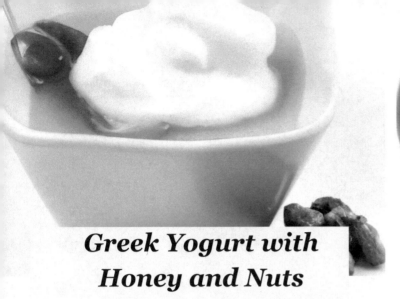

Greek Yogurt with Honey and Nuts

(Greece)

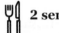 2 servings 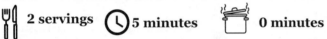 5 minutes 0 minutes

INGREDIENTS

- 1 cup dense Greek yogurt
- 2 tablespoons Greek honey
- 1/4 cup coarsely chopped nuts

DIRECTIONS

Equally, divide the Greek yogurt between two bowls. Drizzle a tablespoon of honey over each serving of yogurt. Sprinkle the chopped nuts over the yogurt. Lightly stir before eating to combine the flavors or enjoy the layers of taste separately, savoring the contrast between the creamy yogurt, the sweetness of the honey, and the crunch of the nuts.

CALORIES	PROTEIN	FATS	FIBRE
180 KCAL	10 G	8 G	1G

Barley Porridge with Fresh Fruit

(Italy)

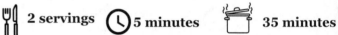 2 servings 5 minutes 35 minutes

INGREDIENTS

- 1 cup pearled barley
- 3 cups water or milk
- 1 apple, diced
- 1/2 cup mixed berries
- 1 teaspoon ground cinnamon
- Honey or maple syrup, to taste

DIRECTIONS

In a medium saucepan, bring the water or milk to a boil. Add the pearled barley and reduce the heat. Cover and simmer for 30-35 minutes or until the barley is tender and has absorbed most of the liquid. Add the diced apple and cinnamon in the last 10 minutes of cooking. Serve the barley warm in bowls, topped with mixed berries and a drizzle of honey or maple syrup for sweetness.

CALORIES	PROTEIN	FATS	FIBRE
250 KCAL	6G	1,5G	10G

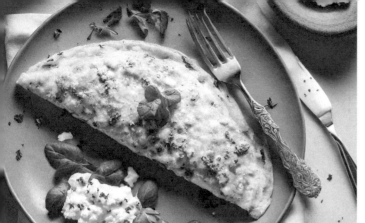

Herb Omelette with Queso Fresco

(Spain)

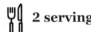 2 servings 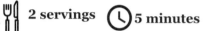 5 minutes   5 minutes

INGREDIENTS

- 4 large eggs
- 1/4 cup milk
- 1/4 cup crumbled queso fresco
- 2 tablespoons mixed fresh herbs (parsley, cilantro, dill), chopped
- 1 tablespoon olive oil
- Salt and black pepper, to taste

DIRECTIONS

Whisk the eggs with the milk, salt, and pepper until smooth. Heat the olive oil in a non-stick skillet over medium heat. Pour in the egg mixture and cook for 1-2 minutes until it begins to set at the edges. Sprinkle the omelet with crumbled queso fresco and chopped fresh herbs. Gently fold it in half and cook for another 1-2 minutes until it is cooked but still soft inside. Serve immediately.

CALORIES	PROTEIN	FATS	FIBRE
220 KCAL	14 G	17G	0 G

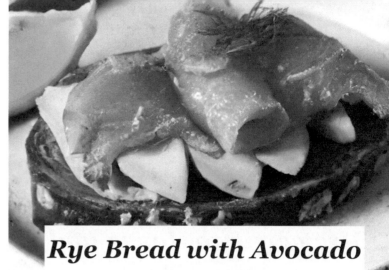

Rye Bread with Avocado and Smoked Salmon

(Portugal)

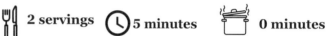 2 servings 5 minutes   0 minutes

INGREDIENTS

- 4 slices of rye bread
- 1 ripe avocado
- 4 slices of smoked salmon
- Juice of 1 lemon
- Salt and black pepper, to taste

DIRECTIONS

Toast the slices of rye bread until they are crispy. Meanwhile, mash the avocado and season it with half lemon juice, salt, and pepper. Spread the mashed avocado evenly over the toasted bread slices. Top each slice with a piece of smoked salmon. Drizzle the remaining lemon juice over the salmon and add a sprinkle of black pepper. Serve immediately to enjoy the freshness of the ingredients.

CALORIES	PROTEIN	FATS	FIBRE
300 KCAL	15G	18G	7G

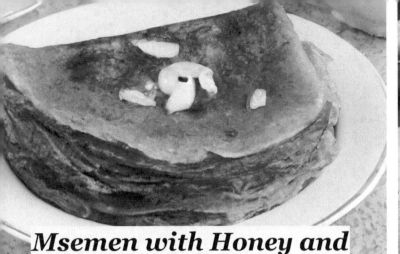

Msemen with Honey and Almonds

(Morocco)

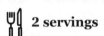 2 servings 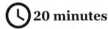 20 minutes 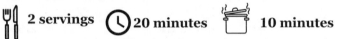 10 minutes

INGREDIENTS

- 1 cup all-purpose flour
- 1/2 cup warm water
- A pinch of salt
- 2 tablespoons melted butter
- 1/4 cup roughly chopped almonds
- Honey, for serving

DIRECTIONS

Mix the flour with salt in a bowl. Gradually add the water, kneading until a smooth and elastic dough forms. Let it rest covered for 10 minutes. Divide the dough into balls. Roll out each ball into a thin sheet, brush with melted butter, and sprinkle with chopped almonds. Fold it several times to form a square. Heat a non-stick pan and cook each semen until golden and crispy on both sides. Serve warm with a generous drizzle of honey on top.

CALORIES	PROTEIN	FATS	FIBRE
350 KCAL	6G	14G	2G

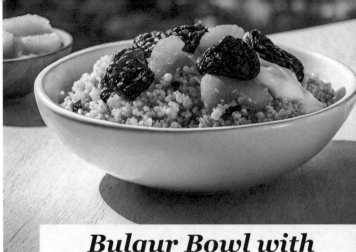

Bulgur Bowl with Yogurt and Dried Fruit

(Cyprus)

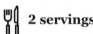 2 servings 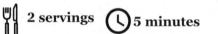 5 minutes 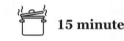 15 minutes

INGREDIENTS

- 1/2 cup bulgur
- 1 cup water
- 1/2 cup dense Greek yogurt
- 2 tablespoons honey
- 1/4 cup mixed nuts, chopped
- 1/4 cup mixed dried fruit (raisins, chopped apricots, dates)

1/2 teaspoon ground cinnamon

DIRECTIONS

Bring water to a boil in a small saucepan; add bulgur and a pinch of salt. Reduce heat, cover, and simmer until the bulgur is tender and has absorbed all the water, about 12-15 minutes. Allow to cool slightly. In serving bowls, evenly distribute the bulgur. Top each portion of bulgur with a dollop of Greek yogurt, then sprinkle with chopped nuts and mixed dried fruit. Finish with a dusting of cinnamon and drizzle with honey before serving for a sweet and nutritious breakfast.

CALORIES	PROTEIN	FATS	FIBRE
400 KCAL	12G	12G	8G

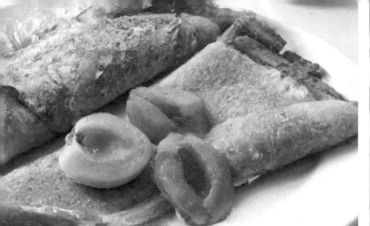

Whole Wheat Crepes with Apricot Compote

(France)

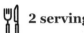 2 servings 10 minutes 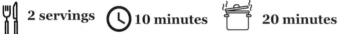 20 minutes

INGREDIENTS

- 1 cup whole wheat flour
- 1 1/2 cups milk
- 2 eggs
- A pinch of salt
- 1 tablespoon olive oil
- 1/2 cup apricot compote

DIRECTIONS

Mix the whole wheat flour, milk, eggs, salt, and olive oil in a bowl until you have a smooth batter. Heat a non-stick pan over medium heat and pour a slight batter into the pan, tilting to spread evenly. Cook for about 2 minutes or until the edges peel off easily, then flip the crepe and cook for another 1-2 minutes. Repeat with the remaining batter. Serve the crepes warm with a spoonful of apricot compote spread over each.

CALORIES 420 KCAL,	PROTEIN 14G	FATS 12G	FIBRE 8G

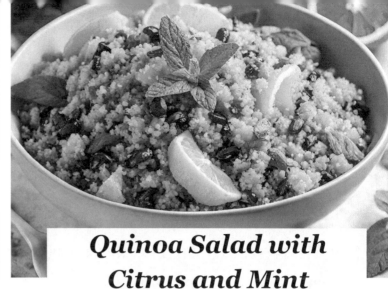

Quinoa Salad with Citrus and Mint

(Greece)

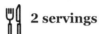 2 servings 10 minutes 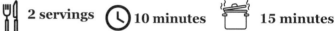 15 minutes

INGREDIENTS

- 1 cup quinoa
- 2 cups water
- 1 orange, segmented
- 1 grapefruit, segmented
- 1/4 cup fresh mint leaves, chopped
- 2 tablespoons extra virgin olive oil
- Salt and black pepper, to taste

DIRECTIONS

Rinse quinoa under cold running water. In a pot, bring water to a boil. Add quinoa and a pinch of salt. Reduce heat, cover, and cook until the quinoa is tender and has absorbed all the water, about 15 minutes. Let cool. In a large bowl, combine cooled quinoa with orange and grapefruit segments, chopped mint, and a drizzle of olive oil, salt, and pepper. Gently mix to combine. Serve the salad cold or at room temperature.

CALORIES 320 KCAL	PROTEIN 8G	FATS 10G	FIBRE 6G

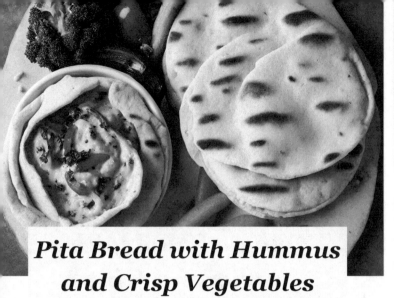

Pita Bread with Hummus and Crisp Vegetables

(Morocco)

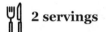 2 servings 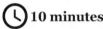 10 minutes 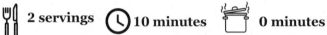 0 minutes

INGREDIENTS

- 2 pita bread rounds
- 1 cup hummus
- 1 carrot, cut into sticks
- 1 cucumber, cut into sticks
- 1/2 red bell pepper, cut into strips
- Lettuce leaves or baby spinach
- 1/4 cup black olives, pitted
- Olive oil, for garnish
- Paprika, for garnish

DIRECTIONS

Open the pita breads and spread them generously with hummus. Evenly distribute the carrot sticks, cucumber sticks, and red bell pepper strips inside each pita. Add a few lettuce leaves or baby spinach and sprinkle with black olives. For a finishing touch, drizzle with olive oil and a dusting of paprika. Serve immediately to enjoy the freshness and crunchiness of the vegetables.

CALORIES	PROTEIN	FATS	FIBRE
310 KCAL	10G	12G	9G

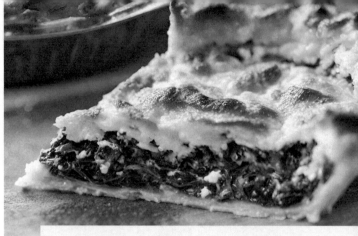

Spinach and Ricotta Savory Pie

(Italy)

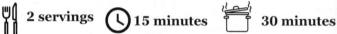 2 servings 15 minutes   30 minutes

INGREDIENTS

- 1 roll of ready-made puff pastry
- 1 cup fresh spinach, washed and chopped
- 1/2 cup ricotta cheese
- 2 eggs
- 1/4 cup grated Parmesan cheese
- Salt and black pepper, to taste
- A pinch of nutmeg

DIRECTIONS

Preheat the oven to 375°F (190°C). Roll out the puff pastry in a baking dish lined with parchment paper. Mix the spinach with ricotta, eggs, Parmesan, salt, pepper, and nutmeg until well combined. Pour the filling onto the puff pastry and fold the edges inwards to close the pie. Bake in the oven for about 30 minutes or until the surface is golden and the puff pastry is crispy. Let it cool for a few minutes before serving.

CALORIES	PROTEIN	FATS	FIBRE
420 KCAL	18G	26G	2G

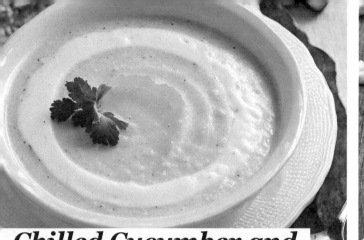

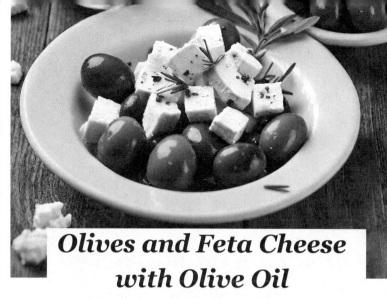

Chilled Cucumber and Yogurt Gazpacho

(Spain)

 2 servings   🕐 15 minutes   🍲 0 minutes

INGREDIENTS

2 large cucumbers, peeled and chopped
1 cup natural Greek yogurt
1 garlic clove, minced
2 tablespoons extra virgin olive oil
1 tablespoon white wine vinegar
Salt and white pepper, to taste
Fresh herbs (dill or mint) for garnish

DIRECTIONS

Place the cucumbers, yogurt, garlic, olive oil, vinegar, salt, and pepper in a blender and blend until smooth. Taste and adjust seasoning if necessary. Chill in the refrigerator for at least 1 hour before serving. Garnish with chopped fresh herbs when serving.

CALORIES 180 KCAL	PROTEIN 9G	FATS 11G	FIBRE 2G

Olives and Feta Cheese with Olive Oil

(Greece)

 2 servings   🕐 5 minutes   🍲 0 minutes

INGREDIENTS

- 1 cup mixed olives, pitted
- 1/2 cup feta cheese, crumbled
- 2 tablespoons extra virgin olive oil
- 1 teaspoon dried oregano
- Freshly ground black pepper, to taste

DIRECTIONS

In a medium bowl, combine the olives and crumbled feta cheese. Drizzle with extra virgin olive oil and sprinkle with dried oregano. Add a twist of freshly ground black pepper for an additional layer of flavor. Gently mix to ensure all the ingredients are well coated. This dish can be served as an appetizer or a healthy morning snack, bringing Mediterranean flavors directly to your table.

CALORIES 250KCAL	PROTEIN 6G	FATS 23G	FIBRE 3G

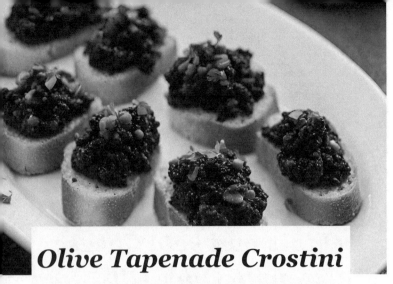

Olive Tapenade Crostini

(France)

 2 servings 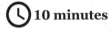 10 minutes 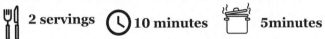 5 minutes

INGREDIENTS

- 1 whole-grain baguette, sliced
- 1/2 cup black olive tapenade
- 1 garlic clove
- 2 tablespoons extra virgin olive oil

DIRECTIONS

Toast the baguette slices under a grill or in a skillet until golden and crispy. Rub lightly one side of each toasted slice with a garlic clove for a subtle flavor. Spread a generous layer of black olive tapenade on each slice and drizzle with a bit of extra virgin olive oil before serving. These crostini offer a perfect balance of intense flavors and are ideal for starting your day with energy or as an appetizer before dinner.

CALORIES	PROTEIN	FATS	FIBRE
290 KCAL	6G	16G	4G

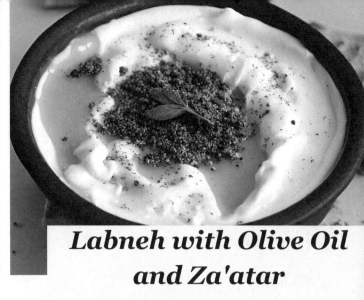

Labneh with Olive Oil and Za'atar

(Morocco)

 2 servings 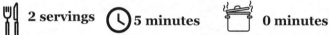 5 minutes 0 minutes

INGREDIENTS

- 1 cup labneh (thick Greek yogurt can be used as a substitute)
- 2 tablespoons extra virgin olive oil
- 1 tablespoon za'atar
- Pita bread for serving

DIRECTIONS

Spread the labneh in a serving bowl and create a well in the center with the back of a spoon. Pour over the olive oil and evenly sprinkle the za'atar. Serve with warm pita bread, perfect for starting your day with a meal that combines rich flavors and creamy textures.

CALORIES	PROTEIN	FATS	FIBRE
150 KCAL	9G	10G	1G

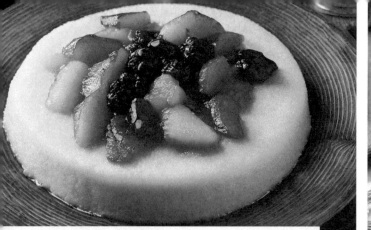

Sweet Polenta with Caramelized Fruit

(Italy)

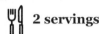 2 servings  5 minutes   15 minutes

INGREDIENTS

- 1/2 cup fine polenta
- 2 cups milk
- 1/4 cup sugar, plus extra for caramelizing the fruit
- 1/2 teaspoon vanilla extract
- 1 apple and 1 pear, sliced
- 1 tablespoon butter
- A pinch of cinnamon

DIRECTIONS

Bring the milk to a boil with a pinch of salt in a medium saucepan. Gradually whisk in the polenta, stirring constantly to avoid lumps. Lower the heat and continue to cook, stirring often, until the polenta becomes creamy, about 10-15 minutes. Stir in the sugar and vanilla extract. In a skillet, melt the butter over medium heat and add the slices of apple and pear, sprinkling them with a bit of sugar and cinnamon. Cook, stirring occasionally, until the fruit is caramelized and tender. Serve the warm polenta topped with the caramelized fruit.

CALORIES 350 KCAL	PROTEIN 8G	FATS 9G	FIBRE 4G

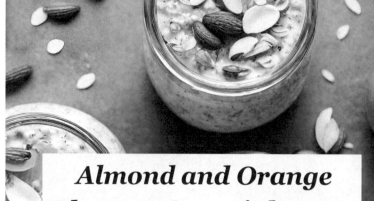

Almond and Orange Blossom Overnight Oats

(Marocco)

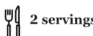 2 servings 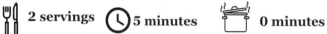 5 minutes   0 minutes

INGREDIENTS

- 1 cup rolled oats
- 1½ cups almond milk
- 2 tbsp almond butter
- 1 tbsp orange blossom water
- 1 tbsp honey or maple syrup
- 1 orange, zest, and segments
- A handful of sliced almonds
- A pinch of salt

DIRECTIONS

Mix the oats, almond milk, almond butter, orange blossom water, honey or maple syrup, and a pinch of salt in a bowl. Cover this mixture and let it sit in the refrigerator overnight to let the oats soften and the flavors meld together. Before serving, stir the mixture well; if it seems too thick, you can adjust the consistency by adding a little more almond milk. Finally, garnish with fresh orange zest, orange segments, and a sprinkle of sliced almonds for added texture and flavor.

CALORIES 300 KCAL;	PROTEIN 8G	FATS 9G	FIBRE 6G

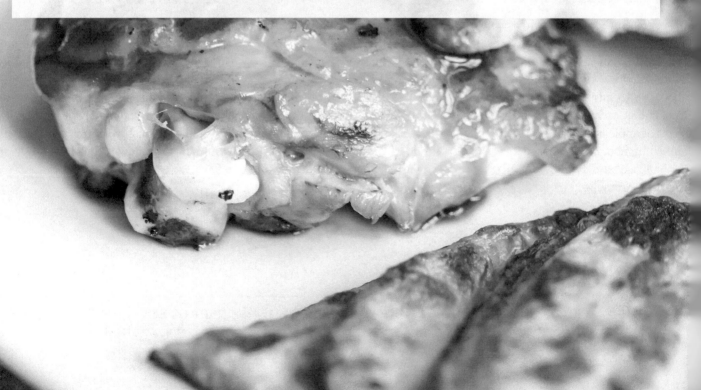

Chicken
Recipes

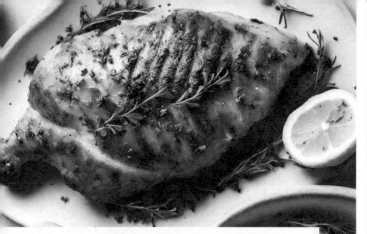

Lemon and Oregano Chicken

(Greece)

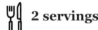 2 servings 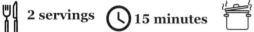 15 minutes 45 minutes

INGREDIENTS

- 2 chicken breasts (about 1 pound)
- 1/4 cup extra virgin olive oil
- Juice of 2 lemons
- 2 cloves garlic, chopped
- 1 tablespoon fresh oregano, chopped
- Salt and black pepper, to taste

DIRECTIONS

Mix olive oil, lemon juice, garlic, oregano, salt, and pepper in a bowl. Marinate the chicken breasts in this mixture for at least 1 hour in the refrigerator. Preheat the oven to 375°F (190°C). Arrange the chicken and marinade in a baking dish and bake for 45 minutes or until the chicken is well-cooked and golden. Serve the chicken hot, drizzled with the cooking juice.

CALORIES 350 KCAL	PROTEIN 40G	FATS 18G	FIBRE 0G

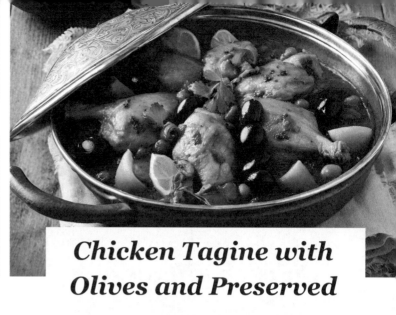

Chicken Tagine with Olives and Preserved

(Morocco)

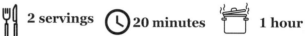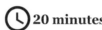 2 servings 20 minutes 1 hour

INGREDIENTS

- 2 chicken thighs (about 1 pound)
- 1/4 cup green olives, pitted
- 1 preserved lemon, sliced
- 1 medium onion, sliced
- 2 cloves garlic, chopped
- 1 teaspoon ground cumin
- 1 teaspoon ground coriander
- 1/2 teaspoon turmeric
- 1/4 teaspoon cayenne pepper
- 2 tablespoons extra virgin olive oil
- 1 cup chicken broth
- Salt and black pepper, to taste
- Fresh coriander, chopped for garnish

DIRECTIONS

Heat the oil and sauté onion and garlic in a tagine or heavy casserole. Add the spices and chicken thighs, browning them. Add the broth, olives, and preserved lemons. Cover and cook on low heat for about 1 hour or until the chicken is tender. Serve the tagine garnished with fresh coriander.

CALORIES 410 KCAL	PROTEIN 35G	FATS 24G	FIBRE 2G

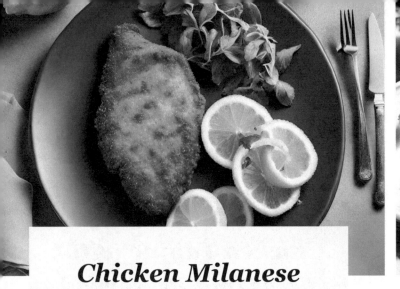

Chicken Milanese

(Italy)

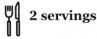 2 servings   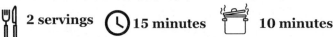 15 minutes   10 minutes

INGREDIENTS

- 2 chicken breasts, flattened
- 1/2 cup flour
- 2 eggs, beaten
- 1 cup breadcrumbs
- Salt and black pepper, to taste
- 4 tablespoons olive oil for frying
- Lemon wedges to serve

DIRECTIONS

Season the chicken breasts with salt and pepper. Dredge in flour, dip in beaten egg, and coat in breadcrumbs pressing to adhere well. In a skillet, heat the oil and fry the chicken over medium-high heat until golden on both sides, about 5 minutes per side. Serve hot with lemon wedges.

CALORIES	PROTEIN	FATS	FIBRE
520 KCAL	35G	28G	1G

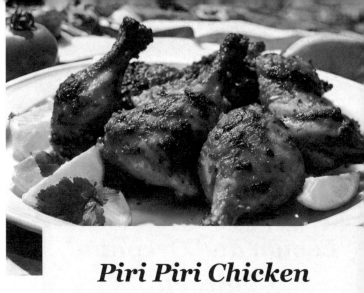

Piri Piri Chicken

(Portugal)

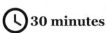 2 servings   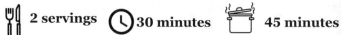 30 minutes    45 minutes

INGREDIENTS

- 2 chicken thighs (about 1 pound)
- 2 tablespoons piri piri sauce
- 2 cloves garlic, chopped
- 1 tablespoon paprika
- Juice of 1 lemon
- 2 tablespoons olive oil
- Salt and black pepper, to taste

DIRECTIONS

Mix piri piri sauce, garlic, paprika, lemon juice, olive oil, salt, and pepper in a bowl. Marinate the chicken thighs in this mixture for at least 2 hours, preferably overnight. Preheat the oven to 375°F (190°C). Arrange the chicken in a baking dish and bake for 45 minutes, until well cooked and the skin is crispy. Serve hot.

CALORIES	PROTEIN	FATS	FIBRE
430 KCAL	35G	32G	0G

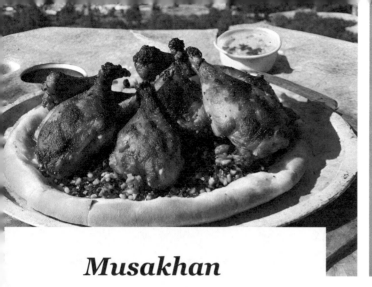

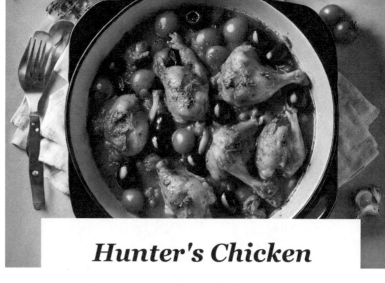

Musakhan

(Palestine)

🍴 2 servings 🕐 20 minutes 🍲 1 hour

INGREDIENTS

- 2 chicken thighs
- 2 large onions, sliced
- 2 tablespoons sumac
- 1/4 cup pine nuts, toasted
- 2 tablespoons olive oil
- Salt and black pepper, to taste
- 2 taboon bread or pita
- Fresh coriander, for garnish

DIRECTIONS

In a skillet, heat the oil and sauté the onions until soft. Add sumac, pine nuts, salt, and pepper. Arrange the chicken on top of the onions and bake in the oven at 375°F (190°C) for about 1 hour, until the chicken is cooked. Serve the chicken and onions on taboon bread garnished with fresh coriander.

Hunter's Chicken

(Italy)

🍴 2 servings 🕐 20 minutes 🍲 1 hour

INGREDIENTS

- 2 chicken thighs
- 1/2 cup red wine
- 1 medium onion, chopped
- 2 cloves garlic, chopped
- 1/2 cup canned tomatoes, chopped
- 1/4 cup black olives, pitted
- 1 tablespoon capers
- 1 sprig of rosemary
- 2 tablespoons extra virgin olive oil
- Salt and black pepper, to taste

DIRECTIONS

In a skillet, heat the oil and brown the chicken. Remove the chicken and, in the same skillet, sauté onion and garlic. Add the red wine and let it evaporate. Add the tomatoes, olives, capers, rosemary, salt, and pepper. Return the chicken to the skillet, cover, and cook over low heat for about 1 hour. Serve hot.

CALORIES 560 KCAL	PROTEIN 38G	FATS 32G	FIBRE 3G

CALORIES 480 KCAL	PROTEIN 38G	FATS 28G	FIBRE 3G

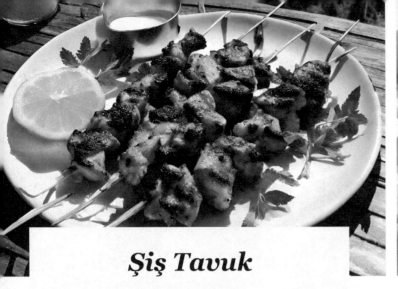

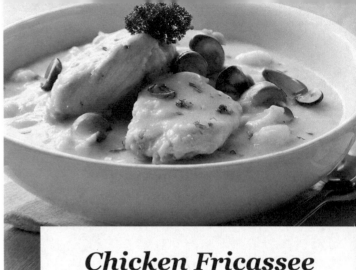

Şiş Tavuk

(Turkey)

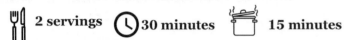 2 servings 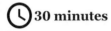 30 minutes 15 minutes

INGREDIENTS

- 1 pound chicken breast, cubed
- 1/2 cup natural yogurt
- Juice of 1 lemon
- 2 cloves garlic, chopped
- 1 teaspoon paprika
- 1/2 teaspoon ground cumin
- Salt and black pepper, to taste
- Olive oil for brushing
- Wooden or metal skewers

DIRECTIONS

Marinate the chicken in yogurt, lemon juice, garlic, paprika, cumin, salt, and pepper for at least 2 hours. Thread the marinated chicken cubes onto skewers. Grill over medium-high heat, brushing with olive oil, until golden and cooked, about 3 minutes per side. Serve hot.

CALORIES	PROTEIN	FATS	FIBRE
310 KCAL	48G	6G	0G

Chicken Fricassee

(France)

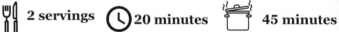 2 servings 20 minutes 45 minutes

INGREDIENTS

- 2 chicken breasts
- 1/2 cup chicken broth
- 1/4 cup white wine
- 1/2 cup heavy cream
- 1 egg yolk
- Juice of 1/2 lemon
- 1/2 cup mushrooms, sliced
- 1/4 cup pearl onions
- 2 tablespoons butter
- Salt and black pepper, to taste
- Fresh parsley, chopped for garnish

DIRECTIONS

In a skillet, cook the chicken breasts in butter until golden. Add mushrooms and pearl onions and cook for a few minutes. Deglaze with white wine, add the broth and cover for 30 minutes. Remove the chicken and add cream, egg yolk, and lemon juice to the skillet, stirring until it thickens. Pour the sauce over the chicken and garnish with parsley.

CALORIES	PROTEIN	FATS	FIBRE
540 KCAL	38G	36G	1G

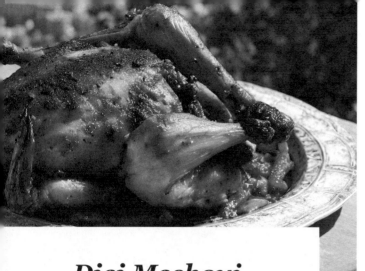

Djej Mechoui

(Algeria)

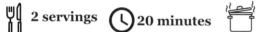 2 servings 20 minutes 🍲 90 minutes

INGREDIENTS

- 1 whole chicken (about 3-4 pounds)
- 4 cloves garlic, finely chopped
- 2 teaspoons paprika
- 1 teaspoon ground cumin
- 1/2 teaspoon chili powder
- 1/4 cup olive oil
- Salt and black pepper, to taste
- 1 lemon, cut into wedges for serving

DIRECTIONS

Mix garlic, paprika, cumin, chili, olive oil, salt, and pepper to prepare a marinade. Evenly spread the marinade over the entire chicken, both inside and out. Marinate for at least 2 hours, preferably overnight. Preheat the oven to 375°F (190°C) and roast the chicken for about 1 hour and 30 minutes, until it is golden and the meat quickly pulls away from the bones. Serve hot with lemon wedges.

CALORIES 650 KCAL	PROTEIN 70G	FATS 36G	FIBRE 0G

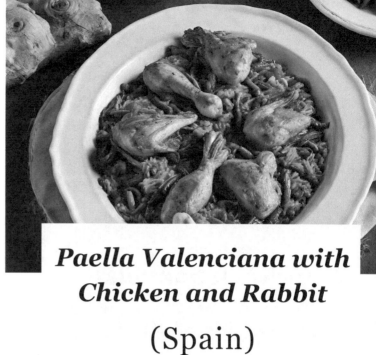

Paella Valenciana with Chicken and Rabbit

(Spain)

 2 servings 30 minutes 🍲 1 hour

INGREDIENTS

- 1/2 pound chicken, cut into pieces
- 1/2 pound rabbit, cut into pieces
- 1 cup short-grain rice
- 2 cups chicken broth
- 1/2 cup green beans, chopped
- 1 medium tomato, chopped
- 1/2 onion, finely chopped
- 1 clove garlic, chopped
- 1/2 teaspoon saffron
- 2 tablespoons extra virgin olive oil
- Salt and black pepper, to taste
- Rosemary sprigs, for garnish

DIRECTIONS

Heat the oil in a paella pan or a large skillet and brown the chicken and rabbit. Add onion, garlic, and green beans, cooking for a few minutes. Stir in tomato and rice, mixing well. Add the broth and saffron, boil, reduce the heat, and cook covered for 20 minutes. Uncover and cook for another 20 minutes until the rice is cooked and the liquid is absorbed. Serve hot, garnished with rosemary.

CALORIES 720 KCAL	PROTEIN 60G	FATS 30G	FIBRE 3G

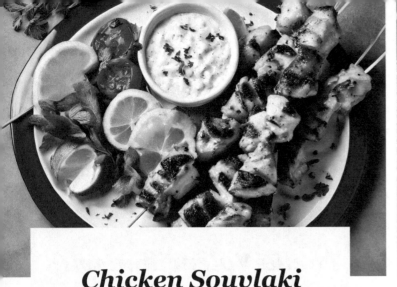

Chicken Souvlaki

(Greece)

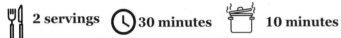 2 servings 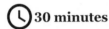 30 minutes 10 minutes

INGREDIENTS

- 1 pound chicken breast, cubed
- 1/4 cup extra virgin olive oil
- Juice of 1 lemon
- 2 cloves garlic, chopped
- 1 tablespoon fresh oregano, chopped
- Salt and black pepper, to taste
- Tzatziki, for serving

DIRECTIONS

Marinate the chicken cubes in olive oil, lemon juice, garlic, oregano, salt, and pepper for at least 2 hours. Thread the chicken cubes onto skewers. Grill over medium-high heat, turning occasionally, until golden and fully cooked, about 5 minutes per side. Serve with tzatziki.

CALORIES	PROTEIN	FATS	FIBRE
400 KCAL	48G	22G	0G

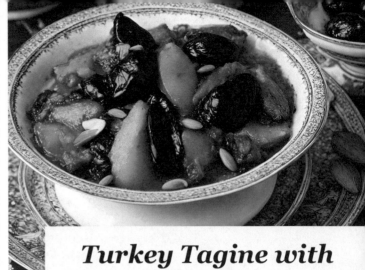

Turkey Tagine with Prunes and Almonds

(Morocco)

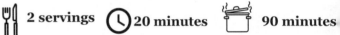 2 servings  20 minutes 90 minutes

INGREDIENTS

- 1 pound turkey thighs
- 1/2 cup dried prunes
- 1/4 cup toasted almonds
- 1 medium onion, chopped
- 2 cloves garlic, chopped
- 1 teaspoon ground cinnamon
- 1/2 teaspoon ground ginger
- 1/4 teaspoon turmeric
- 1/4 teaspoon ground black pepper
- 2 tablespoons olive oil
- 2 cups chicken broth
- Salt, to taste
- Fresh coriander, for garnish

DIRECTIONS

Heat the oil and sauté onion and garlic in a tagine or heavy casserole. Add the turkey and brown on all sides. Incorporate the spices and cook for a couple of minutes. Add the broth and bring to a boil. Reduce the heat, cover, and cook slowly for about 1 hour. Add the prunes and continue cooking for another 30 minutes. Serve the tagine garnished with toasted almonds and fresh coriander.

CALORIES	PROTEIN	FATS	FIBRE
600 KCAL	45G	32G	4G

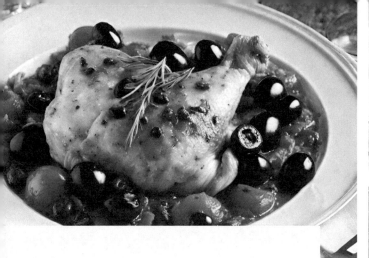

Chicken Provençal

(France, Provence)

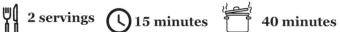 2 servings   15 minutes 40 minutes

INGREDIENTS

- 2 chicken thighs
- 1/2 cup cherry tomatoes, halved
- 1/4 cup black olives, pitted
- 2 tablespoons capers
- 2 cloves garlic, chopped
- 1/4 cup white wine
- 1 tablespoon Herbes de Provence
- 2 tablespoons olive oil
- Salt and black pepper, to taste

DIRECTIONS

In a large skillet, heat the oil and brown the chicken until golden. Add garlic and cook for 1 minute. Deglaze with white wine, then add tomatoes, olives, capers, and Herbes de Provence. Cover and cook over medium-low heat for 40 minutes until the chicken is tender. Serve hot.

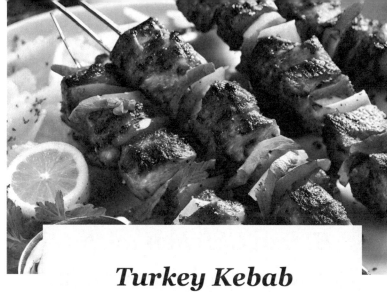

Turkey Kebab

(Turkey)

 2 servings   20 minutes 10 minutes

INGREDIENTS

- 1 pound ground turkey
- 1/4 cup fresh parsley, chopped
- 1/4 cup fresh coriander, chopped
- 1 clove garlic, chopped
- 1 teaspoon paprika
- 1/2 teaspoon ground cumin
- Salt and black pepper, to taste
- Olive oil for grilling

DIRECTIONS

Mix the ground turkey with parsley, coriander, garlic, paprika, cumin, salt, and pepper in a bowl. Form the mixture into skewers and brush them with olive oil. Grill the skewers over medium-high heat, turning occasionally, until they are well cooked and golden, about 5 minutes per side. Serve hot.

CALORIES 460 KCAL	PROTEIN 38G	FATS 28G	FIBRE 2G

CALORIES 320 KCAL	PROTEIN 36G	FATS 18G	FIBRE 1G

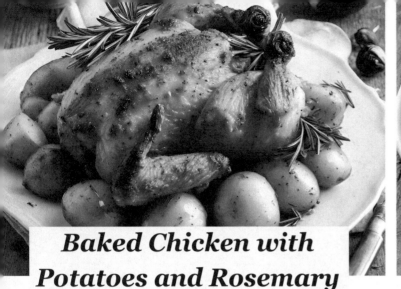

Baked Chicken with Potatoes and Rosemary

(Italy)

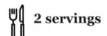 2 servings 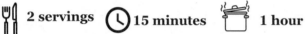 15 minutes 1 hour

INGREDIENTS

- 2 chicken thighs
- 4 medium potatoes, cut into wedges
- 2 sprigs of fresh rosemary
- 4 cloves garlic, whole
- 1/4 cup olive oil
- Salt and black pepper, to taste

DIRECTIONS

Place the chicken thighs, potato wedges, garlic, and rosemary in a baking dish. Season with salt, pepper, and olive oil. Mix well to ensure the seasoning is evenly distributed. Bake in a preheated oven at 400°F (200°C) for 1 hour, until the chicken and potatoes are golden and crispy. Serve hot.

CALORIES 520 KCAL	PROTEIN 35G	FATS 28G	FIBRE 5G

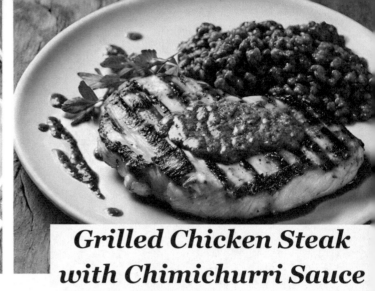

Grilled Chicken Steak with Chimichurri Sauce

(Spain)

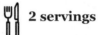 2 servings 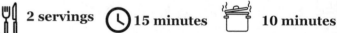 15 minutes 10 minutes

INGREDIENTS

- 2 chicken breast steaks (about 1 pound in total)
- Salt and black pepper, to taste
- Olive oil for grilling
- For the Chimichurri Sauce:
- 1/2 cup fresh parsley, chopped
- 1/4 cup olive oil
- 1/4 cup red wine vinegar
- 2 cloves garlic, chopped
- 1 teaspoon red chili flakes
- 1/2 teaspoon ground cumin
- Salt, to taste

DIRECTIONS

For the sauce, mix parsley, olive oil, vinegar, garlic, chili flakes, cumin, and salt. Let it sit. Season the chicken steaks with salt and pepper. Grill over medium-high heat, brushing with olive oil, until the desired doneness, about 5 minutes per side. Serve the chicken with the chimichurri sauce on top or on the side.

CALORIES 380 KCAL	PROTEIN 40G	FATS 22G	FIBRE 0G

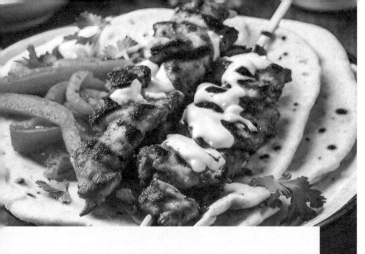

Chicken Shawarma

(Middle East)

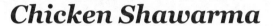 2 servings 20 minutes 10 minutes

INGREDIENTS

- 1 pound chicken breast, thinly sliced
- 2 tablespoons natural yogurt
- 1 tablespoon olive oil
- Juice of 1 lemon
- 2 cloves garlic, chopped
- 1 teaspoon paprika
- 1/2 teaspoon ground cumin
- 1/2 teaspoon ground coriander
- 1/4 teaspoon turmeric
- 1/4 teaspoon ground cinnamon
- Salt and black pepper, to taste
- Pita and salad for serving

DIRECTIONS

Marinate the chicken with yogurt, olive oil, lemon juice, garlic, spices, salt, and pepper for at least 2 hours. Grill or cook in a skillet over medium-high heat until golden and cooked, about 5 minutes per side. Serve the chicken inside pita bread with salad.

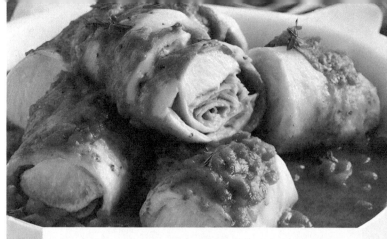

Stuffed Chicken Rolls

(Italy)

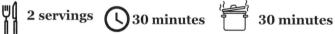 2 servings 30 minutes 30 minutes

INGREDIENTS

- 2 chicken breasts, flattened
- 2 slices of prosciutto
- 2 slices of cheese (e.g., mozzarella or fontina)
- Salt and black pepper, to taste
- 1 cup tomato sauce
- 2 tablespoons olive oil

DIRECTIONS

Place a slice of prosciutto and cheese on each flattened chicken breast. Roll up the chicken around the filling and secure it with toothpicks. Season with salt and pepper. In a skillet, heat the oil and brown the rolls on all sides. Add the tomato sauce and cook covered over medium-low heat for 20-30 minutes. Serve the rolls sliced with the sauce.

CALORIES 330 KCAL	PROTEIN 48G	FATS 9G	FIBRE 1G

CALORIES 490 KCAL	PROTEIN 52G	FATS 24G	FIBRE 2G

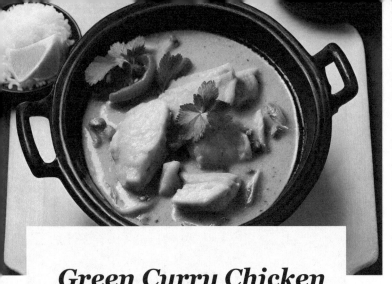

Green Curry Chicken

(Thailand)

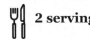 2 servings 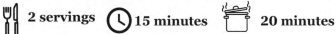 15 minutes 20 minutes

INGREDIENTS

- 1 pound chicken breast, cubed
- 2 tablespoons green curry paste
- 1 can coconut milk (14 ounces)
- 1/2 cup chicken broth
- 1 tablespoon fish sauce
- 1 teaspoon palm sugar or brown sugar
- 1/2 cup bell peppers, sliced
- 1/4 cup Thai basil
- Vegetable oil, for sautéing

DIRECTIONS

Heat a bit of oil in a skillet and sauté the green curry paste for 1 minute. Add the chicken and cook until golden. Mix well in the coconut milk, broth, fish sauce, and sugar. Cook over medium heat for 15 minutes. Add the bell peppers and cook for another 5 minutes. Serve hot, garnished with Thai basil.

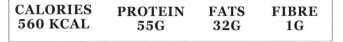

CALORIES 560 KCAL	PROTEIN 55G	FATS 32G	FIBRE 1G

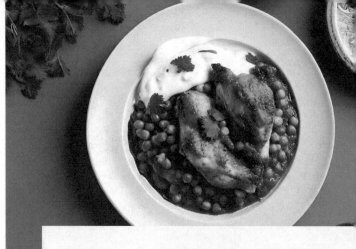

Harissa Chicken with Chickpeas and Yogurt

(Tunisia)

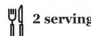 2 servings 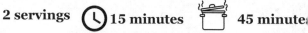 15 minutes 45 minute

INGREDIENTS

- 4 chicken thighs, skin-on, bone-in
- 2 tablespoons harissa paste
- 1 can (14 oz) chickpeas rinsed and drained.
- 1 cup cherry tomatoes
- 1 large onion, sliced
- 2 cloves garlic, minced
- 1 teaspoon cumin seeds
- 1 cup Greek yogurt
- 2 tablespoons olive oil
- Salt and pepper to taste
- Fresh cilantro, chopped, for garnish
- Lemon wedges for serving

DIRECTIONS

Start by preheating your oven to 400°F (200°C). Combine the chicken thighs with harissa paste in a large bowl, ensuring each piece is evenly coated. Set aside to marinate for at least 10 minutes. In a large baking dish, toss the chickpeas, cherry tomatoes, sliced onion, minced garlic, and cumin seeds with olive oil, salt, and pepper. Nestle the marinated chicken thighs among the vegetables. Roast in the preheated oven for about 45 minutes or until the chicken is cooked through and the vegetables are tender. Serve the chicken and vegetables over a bed of Greek yogurt garnished with chopped cilantro. Accompany with lemon wedges on the side for added zest.

CALORIES 550 KCAL	PROTEIN 36G	FATS 32G	FIBRE 6G

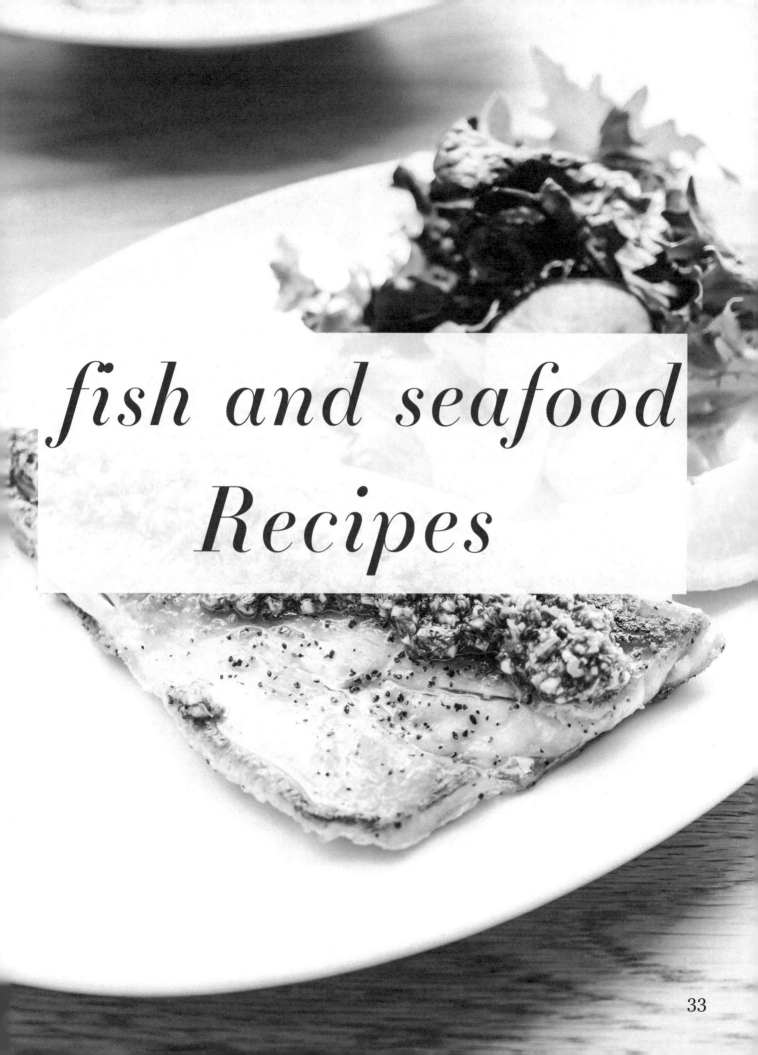

fish and seafood Recipes

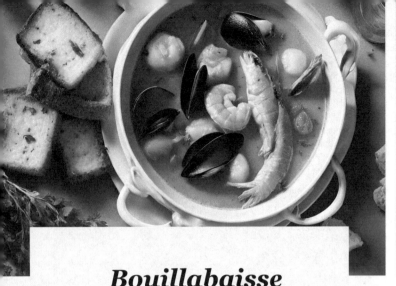
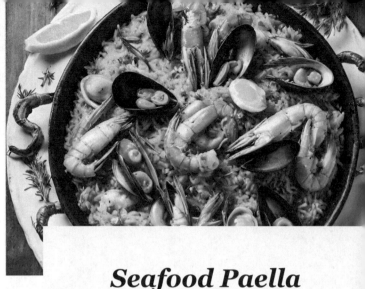

Bouillabaisse

(France, French Riviera)

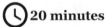 2 servings 20 minutes 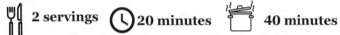 40 minutes

INGREDIENTS

- 10 oz of mixed fish (e.g., scorpion fish, monkfish, cod)
- 4 oz of seafood (e.g., shrimp, mussels)
- 2 cups of fish broth
- 1 ripe tomato, peeled and chopped
- 1/2 onion, finely chopped
- 1 garlic clove, minced
- 1/2 leek, white part only, thinly sliced
- 1 sprig of thyme
- 1 bay leaf
- Saffron, one sachet
- 2 tablespoons of extra virgin olive oil
- Salt and black pepper, to taste
- Croutons
- Rouille, for serving

DIRECTIONS

Heat the oil in a casserole and sauté the onion, garlic, and leek until soft. Add the tomatoes, thyme, bay leaf, and saffron; cook for a few minutes. Pour in the fish broth, bring to a boil, and simmer for 20 minutes. Add the fish and seafood to the broth and cook for another 15-20 minutes until fully cooked. Serve the bouillabaisse with croutons and rouille on the side.

CALORIES	PROTEIN	FATS	FIBRE
310 KCAL	40G	14G	2G

Seafood Paella

(Spain, Valencia)

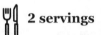 2 servings 30 minutes 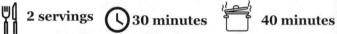 40 minutes

INGREDIENTS

- 1 cup of paella or Arborio rice
- 8 oz of various types of seafood (shrimp, mussels, clams)
- 1/2 cup of frozen peas
- 2 medium tomatoes, chopped
- 1/2 onion, finely chopped
- 1 garlic clove, minced
- 1/2 red bell pepper, diced
- 4 cups of fish broth
- 1/2 teaspoon of saffron
- 1/2 teaspoon of sweet paprika
- 2 tablespoons of extra virgin olive oil
- Salt and black pepper, to taste

DIRECTIONS

Begin by heating the oil in a wide pan and sauté onion, garlic, and bell pepper until soft. Add the rice and toast it slightly before adding the tomatoes, saffron, and paprika. Pour the fish broth and let the rice cook, absorbing the liquid, then add the seafood and peas. Cover and cook until the seafood is fully cooked and the rice is tender. Serve the paella hot, garnishing with lemon slices.

CALORIES	PROTEIN	FATS	FIBRE
560 KCAL	35G	10G	3G

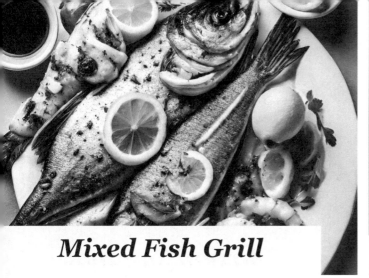

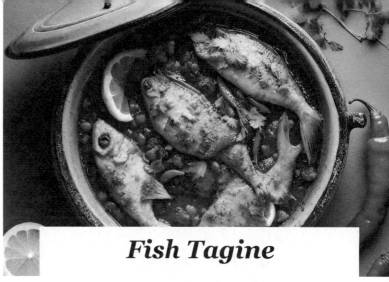

Mixed Fish Grill

Fish Tagine

(Italy)

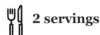 2 servings 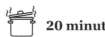 15 minutes 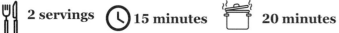 20 minutes

(Morocco)

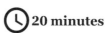 2 servings 20 minutes 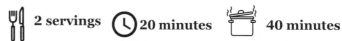 40 minutes

INGREDIENTS

- 8 oz of fresh fish (e.g., sea bass, gilthead seabream)
- 6 cleaned squids
- 2 tablespoons of extra virgin olive oil
- 1 lemon, sliced
- Sea salt and black pepper, to taste
- Fresh parsley, chopped for garnishing

INGREDIENTS

- 8 oz of fish fillet (e.g., cod, tilapia)
- 1 medium potato, cubed
- 1 carrot, sliced
- 1/2 onion, sliced
- 2 tomatoes, chopped
- 2 garlic cloves, minced
- 1 teaspoon of ground cumin
- 1 teaspoon of ground coriander
- 1/2 teaspoon of chili powder
- 2 tablespoons of olive oil
- 1/2 cup of water
- Salt and black pepper, to taste
- Fresh cilantro for garnishing

DIRECTIONS

Heat the grill to medium-high. Season the fish and squids with oil, salt, and pepper. Grill the fish for about 4-5 minutes per side and the squids for 2 minutes per side until they are well-cooked and have a golden crust. Serve immediately with lemon slices and a sprinkle of fresh parsley.

DIRECTIONS

In a tagine or a heavy pot, sauté onion and garlic in oil until golden. Add spices, then potatoes and carrots, covering with water. Cook until the vegetables start to become tender. Add the fish and tomatoes, cover, and simmer until the fish is cooked. Serve garnished with fresh cilantro.

CALORIES 300 KCAL	PROTEIN 45G	FATS 12G	FIBRE 0G

CALORIES 380 KCAL	PROTEIN 35G	FATS 18G	FIBRE 4G

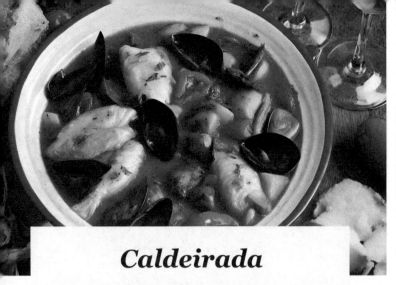

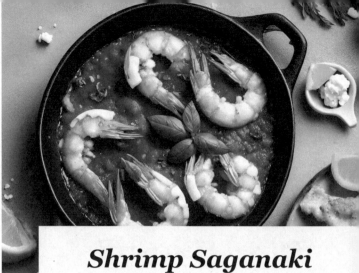

Caldeirada

(Portugal)

🍴 2 servings 🕐 20 minutes 🍲 35 minutes

INGREDIENTS

- 10 oz of mixed fish (e.g., cod, gilthead seabream, scorpionfish)
- 2 medium potatoes, sliced
- 1 large onion, sliced
- 1 red bell pepper, cut into strips
- 2 tomatoes, peeled and chopped
- 2 garlic cloves, minced
- 1/2 cup of white wine
- 1 bay leaf
- 2 tablespoons of extra virgin olive oil
- Salt and black pepper, to taste
- Fresh parsley, chopped for garnishing

DIRECTIONS

In a large pot, sauté onion and garlic in oil. Add potatoes, bell pepper, tomatoes, bay leaf, and a pinch of salt and pepper. Pour in the wine and a bit of water to cover the vegetables. Bring to a boil, reduce heat, and simmer until the potatoes are tender. Add the fish, cover, and cook for another 10-12 minutes. Serve hot, garnished with fresh parsley.

CALORIES	PROTEIN	FATS	FIBRE
420 KCAL	38G	14G	5G

Shrimp Saganaki

(Greece)

🍴 2 servings 🕐 15 minutes 🍲 25 minutes

INGREDIENTS

- 8 oz of shrimp, peeled and deveined
- 1 large tomato, chopped
- 1/2 onion, finely chopped
- 2 garlic cloves, minced
- 1/2 cup of feta cheese, crumbled
- 1/4 cup of white wine
- 1 teaspoon of smoked paprika
- 2 tablespoons of extra virgin olive oil
- Salt and black pepper, to taste
- Fresh parsley, chopped for garnishing

DIRECTIONS

Heat oil in a skillet and sauté onion and garlic until golden. Add shrimp and cook until they turn pink. Pour in the wine and let it evaporate. Add the tomato and paprika, and cook for a few minutes. Season with salt and pepper. Sprinkle with feta and let it cook until the cheese starts to melt. Serve hot, garnished with parsley.

CALORIES	PROTEIN	FATS	FIBRE
350 KCAL	25G	20G	2G

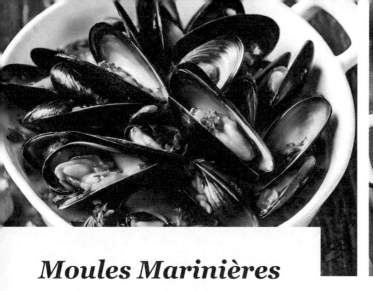

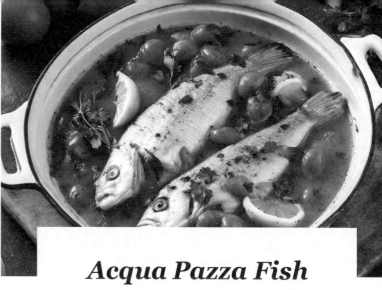

Moules Marinières

(France, Brittany)

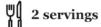 2 servings 10 minutes 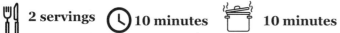 10 minutes

INGREDIENTS

- 2 lbs of mussels, cleaned
- 1/2 cup of dry white wine
- 1/2 onion, finely chopped
- 2 garlic cloves, minced
- 2 tablespoons of fresh parsley, chopped
- 2 tablespoons of butter
- Salt and black pepper, to taste

DIRECTIONS

In a large pot, melt the butter and sauté the onion and garlic until translucent. Add the mussels, pour in the white wine, and cover. Cook for about 5-7 minutes or until all the mussels have opened. Discard any that remain closed. Season with salt and pepper and mix with the chopped parsley. Serve immediately with plenty of sauce and crusty bread for dipping.

CALORIES	PROTEIN	FATS	FIBRE
380 KCAL	24G	18G	0G

Acqua Pazza Fish

(Italy)

 2 servings 15 minutes 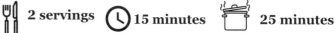 25 minutes

INGREDIENTS

- 2 fillets of sea bream or sea bass, about 6 oz each
- 1 large tomato, chopped
- 1/2 onion, thinly sliced
- 2 garlic cloves, sliced
- 1/2 cup of white wine
- 2 tablespoons of extra virgin olive oil
- 1/4 cup of water
- Salt and black pepper, to taste
- Fresh parsley, chopped for garnishing

DIRECTIONS

Heat the oil and sauté onion and garlic in a wide pan until golden. Add the tomatoes and cook for a few minutes. Place the fish fillets in the pan, pour the wine and water, and cover. Let it cook on medium-low heat for about 20 minutes or until the fish is cooked. Serve garnished with fresh parsley.

CALORIES	PROTEIN	FATS	FIBRE
290 KCAL	35G	12G	1G

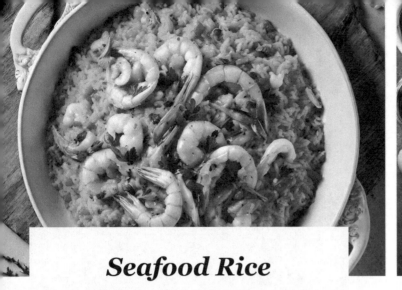
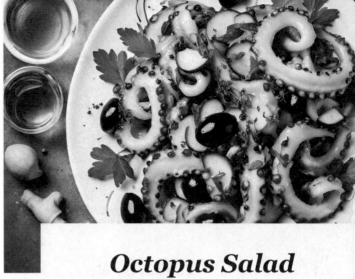

Seafood Rice

(Portugal)

🍴 2 servings 🕐 20 minutes 🍲 40 minutes

INGREDIENTS

- 1 cup of long-grain rice
- 8 oz of mixed seafood (shrimp, clams, mussels)
- 1/2 red bell pepper, diced
- 1/2 onion, finely chopped
- 2 garlic cloves, minced
- 1 large tomato, chopped
- 2 tablespoons of extra virgin olive oil
- 2 cups of fish broth
- 1/2 teaspoon of paprika
- Salt and black pepper, to taste
- Fresh parsley, chopped for garnishing

DIRECTIONS

Heat oil in a pot and sauté onion, garlic, and bell pepper until soft. Add the tomato and paprika and cook for a few minutes. Add the rice and lightly toast it. Pour in the fish broth, bring to a boil, and then reduce the heat. After 10 minutes, add the seafood, cover, and cook until the rice is tender and the seafood is cooked. Serve garnished with fresh parsley.

CALORIES	PROTEIN	FATS	FIBRE
480 KCAL	30G	12G	2G

Octopus Salad

(Greece)

🍴 2 servings 🕐 15 minutes 🍲 90 minutes

INGREDIENTS

- 1 medium octopus, cleaned (about 1 lb)
- 1 cucumber, sliced into half-moons
- 1/2 red onion, thinly sliced
- 1/2 cup of Kalamata olives, pitted
- 2 tablespoons of extra virgin olive oil
- 1 lemon, juiced
- Salt and black pepper, to taste
- Fresh parsley, chopped for garnishing

DIRECTIONS

Cook the octopus in boiling water until tender, about 1 hour and 30 minutes. Let it cool, then cut it into pieces. Combine the octopus with cucumber, onion, olives, olive oil, lemon juice, salt, and pepper in a large bowl. Mix well and refrigerate for at least 30 minutes before serving. Garnish with fresh parsley.

CALORIES	PROTEIN	FATS	FIBRE
310 KCAL	45G	10G	3G

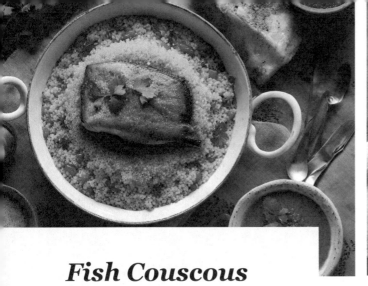
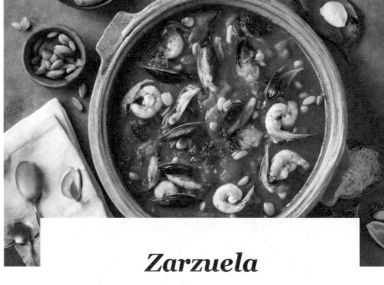

Fish Couscous

(Tunisia)

 2 servings 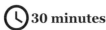 30 minutes 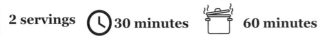 60 minutes

INGREDIENTS

- 1 cup of couscous
- 8 oz of fish fillet of your choice (e.g., cod, sea bream)
- 1 carrot, diced
- 1 zucchini, diced
- 1/2 onion, finely chopped
- 1 garlic clove, minced
- 1/2 cup of cooked chickpeas
- 1/2 teaspoon of harissa (chili paste)
- 1/2 teaspoon of ground cumin
- 1/2 teaspoon of ground coriander
- 2 tablespoons of extra virgin olive oil
- 2 cups of fish broth
- Salt and black pepper, to taste
- Fresh cilantro, chopped for garnishing

DIRECTIONS

In a pot, sauté onion and garlic in oil until golden. Add carrot, zucchini, chickpeas, harissa, cumin, and coriander, and mix well. Pour in the broth and bring to a boil. Add the couscous and reduce the heat. Place the fish fillets on top of the couscous, cover, and cook on low heat until the fish is cooked and the couscous has absorbed the broth, about 15 minutes. Serve garnished with fresh cilantro.

CALORIES 510 KCAL	PROTEIN 35G	FATS 14G	FIBRE 6G

Zarzuela

(Spain, Catalonia)

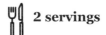 2 servings 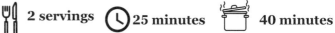 25 minutes 40 minutes

INGREDIENTS

- 8 oz of mixed fish and seafood (e.g., shrimp, clams, squid)
- 1/2 cup of tomato sauce
- 1/2 onion, finely chopped
- 2 garlic cloves, minced
- 1/4 cup of white wine
- 1/2 teaspoon of sweet paprika
- A pinch of saffron
- 2 tablespoons of extra virgin olive oil
- 1/4 cup of water or fish broth
- Salt and black pepper, to taste
- Fresh parsley, chopped for garnishing
- Toasted almonds, chopped for garnishing

DIRECTIONS

In a wide pan, heat the oil and sauté onion and garlic. Add the tomato sauce, wine, paprika, saffron, and some water or broth. Bring to a gentle boil. Add the seafood and cook covered until fully cooked. Serve garnished with parsley and toasted almonds.

CALORIES 420 KCAL	PROTEIN 40G	FATS 16G	FIBRE 3G

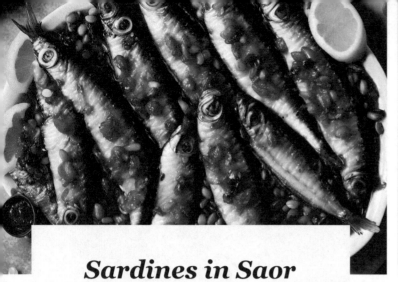

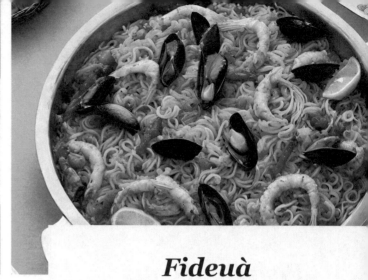

Sardines in Saor

(Italy, Venice)

 2 servings 🕐 20 minutes 🍲 30 minutes

INGREDIENTS

- 8 fresh sardines, cleaned
- 1/2 cup of flour for dredging
- 1/4 cup of extra virgin olive oil
- 1 large onion, thinly sliced
- 1/3 cup of white wine vinegar
- 2 tablespoons of pine nuts
- 2 tablespoons of raisins
- Salt and black pepper, to taste
- Fresh parsley, chopped for garnishing

DIRECTIONS

Dredge the sardines in flour, shaking off the excess. In a pan, heat the oil and fry the sardines until they are golden on both sides. Set aside. In the same pan, add the onion and cook until translucent. Add the vinegar, pine nuts, and raisins. Simmer until the liquid is reduced by half. Pour the saor over the sardines. Let rest for at least 4 hours; it's better if overnight. Serve at room temperature, garnished with parsley.

CALORIES 560 KCAL	PROTEIN 25G	FATS 40G	FIBRE 2G

Fideuà

(Spain, Valencia)

 2 servings 🕐 15 minutes 🍲 30 minutes

INGREDIENTS

- 1/2 lb of short noodle-like pasta
- 8 oz of mixed seafood (shrimp, squid, mussels)
- 1/2 onion, finely chopped
- 1 garlic clove, minced
- 1/2 red bell pepper, diced
- 1/2 cup of tomato sauce
- 2 cups of fish broth
- 1/2 teaspoon of saffron
- 2 tablespoons of extra virgin olive oil
- Salt and black pepper, to taste

DIRECTIONS

In a paellera or a wide pan, sauté onion, garlic, and bell pepper in oil until soft. Add the pasta and lightly toast it. Pour in the tomato sauce and fish broth. Add saffron, salt, and pepper. Cook on medium heat without stirring until the pasta is almost done. Add the seafood and cook until ready. Let rest for a few minutes before serving.

CALORIES 610 KCAL	PROTEIN 25G	FATS 22G	FIBRE 3G

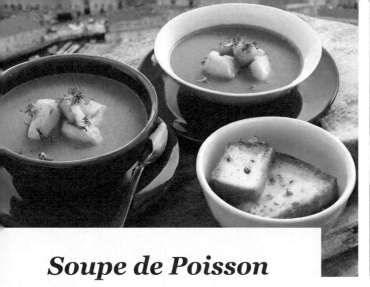

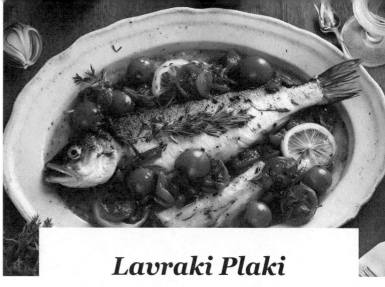

Soupe de Poisson

(France, Marseille)

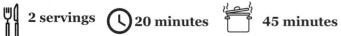 2 servings 20 minutes 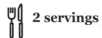 45 minutes

INGREDIENTS

- 1 lb mixed fish (e.g., scorpionfish, cod, monkfish)
- 2 medium tomatoes, chopped
- 1 medium onion, finely chopped
- 1 carrot, diced
- 1 celery stalk, diced
- 2 garlic cloves, minced
- 1/2 cup white wine
- 2 tablespoons extra virgin olive oil
- 4 cups fish stock
- 1 bay leaf
- A pinch of saffron
- Salt and black pepper, to taste
- Rouille and toasted bread slices, for serving

DIRECTIONS

In a large pot, heat the oil and sauté the onion, carrot, celery, and garlic until soft. Add the tomatoes, fish pieces, white wine, fish stock, bay leaf, and saffron. Bring to a boil, then reduce heat and simmer for about 45 minutes. Remove the bay leaf and blend the soup to achieve a smooth consistency. Season with salt and pepper. Serve hot, accompanied by rouille spread on toasted bread slices.

CALORIES 360 KCAL	PROTEIN 40G	FATS 12G	FIBRE 3G

Lavraki Plaki

(Greece)

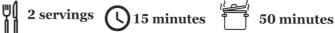 2 servings 15 minutes 50 minutes

INGREDIENTS

- 2 sea bass (about 1 lb each), cleaned and scaled
- 2 large tomatoes, sliced
- 1 large onion, thinly sliced
- 2 medium potatoes, thinly sliced
- 4 garlic cloves, sliced
- 1/2 cup extra virgin olive oil
- 1 lemon, sliced
- Salt and black pepper, to taste
- 1/2 cup water or fish broth
- Fresh parsley, chopped for garnish

DIRECTIONS

Layer the potatoes, tomatoes, onion, and garlic in a baking dish, creating an even base. Place the sea bass on top of the vegetables and season with oil, salt, and pepper. Top with lemon slices. Pour the water or broth into the dish. Cover with aluminum foil and bake in a preheated oven at 375°F (190°C) for about 50 minutes. Uncover and broil for another 5-10 minutes. Garnish with fresh parsley before serving.

CALORIES 550 KCAL	PROTEIN 55G	FATS 28G	FIBRE 4G

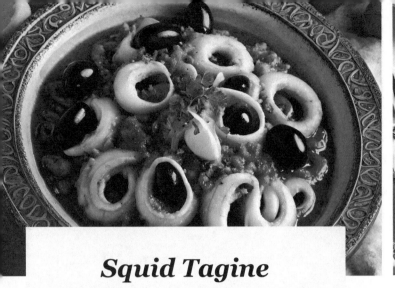

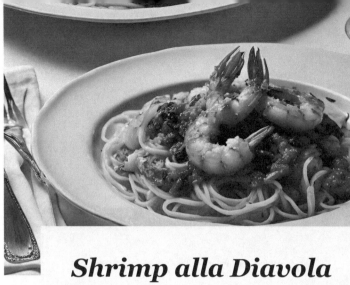

Squid Tagine

(Morocco)

🍴 2 servings 🕐 20 minutes 🍲 60 minutes

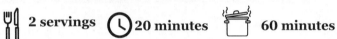

INGREDIENTS

- 1 lb squid, cleaned and cut into rings
- 2 large tomatoes, peeled and chopped
- 1/2 onion, finely chopped
- 2 cloves of garlic, minced
- 1 teaspoon paprika
- 1/2 teaspoon ground cumin
- 1/4 teaspoon chili powder
- 2 tablespoons extra virgin olive oil
- 1/2 cup water or fish broth
- Salt and black pepper, to taste
- Fresh cilantro, chopped for garnish
- Lemon wedges for serving

DIRECTIONS

Heat the oil and sauté the onion and garlic until golden in a tagine or a heavy casserole. Add the squid, tomatoes, paprika, cumin, chili, salt, and pepper. Mix well, then add the water or broth. Cover and cook over low heat for about 60 minutes until the squid is tender. Serve garnished with fresh cilantro and accompanied by lemon wedges.

CALORIES	PROTEIN	FATS	FIBRE
320 KCAL	30G	14G	2G

Shrimp alla Diavola

(Italy, Sicily)

🍴 2 servings 🕐 15 minutes 🍲 10 minutes

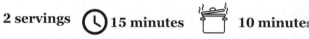

INGREDIENTS

- 1 lb shrimp, peeled and deveined
- 2 cloves of garlic, minced
- 1 red chili, finely chopped
- 1/2 cup tomato sauce
- 1/4 cup white wine
- 2 tablespoons extra virgin olive oil
- Salt and black pepper, to taste
- Fresh parsley, chopped for garnish
- Al dente pasta, for serving

DIRECTIONS

In a skillet, heat the oil and sauté the garlic and chili until the garlic is golden. Add the shrimp and cook until they turn pink. Deglaze with white wine, then add the tomato sauce. Cook for about 5 minutes until the sauce thickens. Serve the hot shrimp over a bed of al dente pasta, garnished with fresh parsley.

CALORIES	PROTEIN	FATS	FIBRE
380 KCAL	48G	16G	1G

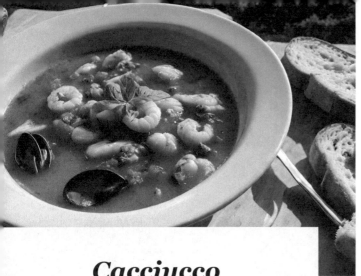

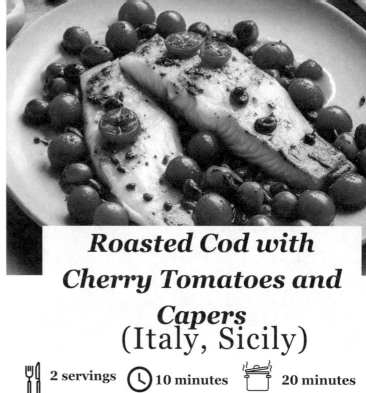

Cacciucco

(Italy, Tuscany)

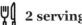 2 servings 30 minutes 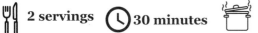 90 minutes

INGREDIENTS

- 1 lb mixed seafood (e.g., squid, clams, mussels, scorpionfish)
- 1/2 cup tomato sauce
- 1/2 onion, finely chopped
- 2 cloves of garlic, minced
- 1/4 cup red wine
- 2 tablespoons extra virgin olive oil
- 1 red chili, chopped
- 1 liter fish broth
- Salt and black pepper, to taste
- Fresh parsley, chopped for garnish
- Toasted bread slices for serving

DIRECTIONS

Heat the oil and sauté the onion, garlic, and chili in a large pot. Add the mixed seafood and cook for a few minutes. Deglaze with red wine, then add the tomato sauce and fish broth. Simmer on low heat for about 1 hour and 30 minutes. Serve the cacciucco hot over toasted bread slices, garnished with fresh parsley.

CALORIES	PROTEIN	FATS	FIBRE
450 KCAL	55G	18G	2G

Roasted Cod with Cherry Tomatoes and Capers

(Italy, Sicily)

2 servings 10 minutes 20 minutes

INGREDIENTS

- 4 cod fillets
- 2 cups cherry tomatoes, halved
- 3 tablespoons capers, rinsed
- 4 garlic cloves, thinly sliced
- 1/4 cup extra virgin olive oil
- 1 lemon, zest and juice
- Fresh basil leaves for garnish
- Salt and freshly ground black pepper to taste

DIRECTIONS

Preheat your oven to 400°F (200°C) and place the cod fillets in a large baking dish in a single layer. Scatter cherry tomatoes, capers, and sliced garlic around and on top of the fillets. Generously drizzle with extra virgin olive oil, sprinkle with lemon zest, and season with salt and pepper to your liking. Roast everything for about 20 minutes, until the cod is flaky and fully cooked, and the tomatoes softened. Finish by squeezing fresh lemon juice over the dish and garnishing with fresh basil leaves to serve.

CALORIES	PROTEIN	FATS	FIBRE
280 KCAL	23G	15G	2G

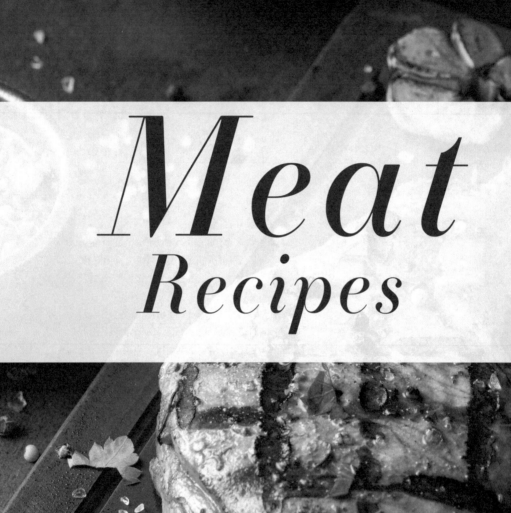

Meat
Recipes

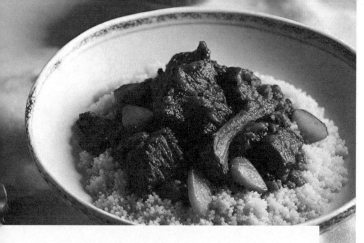

Moroccan Lamb Stew

(Morocco)

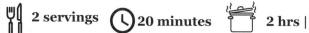 2 servings 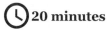 20 minutes 2 hrs |

INGREDIENTS

- 1 lb lamb, cubed
- 1/2 cup dried prunes
- 1/4 cup almonds
- 1 large onion, chopped
- 2 cloves garlic, minced
- 2 tsp cinnamon
- 1 tsp saffron
- 2 tbsp olive oil
- 2 cups beef broth
- Salt and pepper

DIRECTIONS

Heat the olive oil in a large saucepan and brown the lamb cubes on all sides. Add the onion and garlic, sautéing until translucent. Season with cinnamon and saffron, mixing well to coat the lamb. Pour the beef broth to cover the lamb, boil, then reduce heat and simmer covered for about 1.5 hours until the lamb is tender. Add the dried prunes and almonds and cook for another 30 minutes. Ensure the meat is tender and the sauce has thickened before serving.

CALORIES 710 KCAL	PROTEIN 48G	FATS 36G	FIBRE 5G

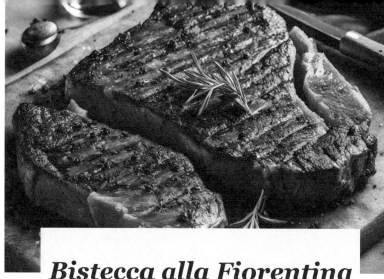

Bistecca alla Fiorentina

(Italy)

2 servings 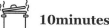 10 minutes 10minutes

INGREDIENTS

- 1 Fiorentina steak, 2 lb and about 2 inches thick
- Coarse salt and freshly ground black pepper
- 2 tbsp extra virgin olive oil

DIRECTIONS

Let the steak reach room temperature before cooking. Heat a grill or grill pan to high. Season both sides of the steak generously with coarse salt and black pepper. Grill the steak for 5 minutes on each side for rare, turning only once. Rest the steak for a few minutes before slicing it against the grain. Serve hot, drizzled with extra virgin olive oil.

CALORIES 850 KCAL	PROTEIN 92G	FATS 40G	FIBRE 0G

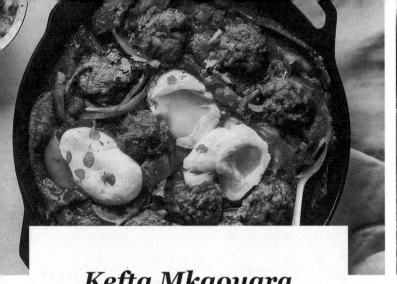

Kefta Mkaouara

(Morocco)

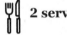 2 servings 20 minutes 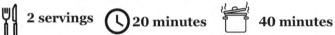 40 minutes

INGREDIENTS

- 1 lb ground beef or lamb
- 1 can (14 oz) crushed tomatoes
- 1 medium onion, finely chopped
- 2 cloves garlic, minced
- 2 tbsp fresh cilantro, chopped
- 1 tsp paprika
- 1 tsp cumin
- 1/2 tsp chili powder
- 4 large eggs
- Salt and black pepper, to taste
- 2 tbsp olive oil

DIRECTIONS

Mix the ground meat with half the chopped onion, garlic, cilantro, paprika, cumin, chili, salt, and pepper. Form small meatballs and set aside. In a pan, heat the oil and sauté the remaining onion until translucent. Add the crushed tomatoes, salt, and pepper, and cook over medium heat for about 10 minutes. Place the meatballs in the sauce, cover, and simmer for 30 minutes. Make small wells between the meatballs and crack an egg into each, cover again, and cook until the eggs are just set. Serve hot with Moroccan bread or pita.

CALORIES	PROTEIN	FATS	FIBRE
650 KCAL	40G	45G	4G

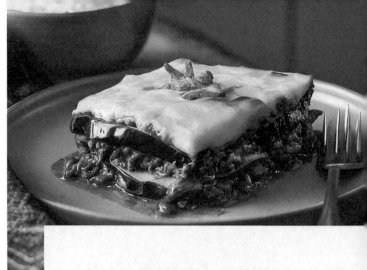

Moussaka

(Greece)

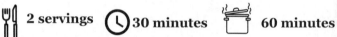 2 servings 30 minutes 60 minutes

INGREDIENTS

- 1 lb eggplant, sliced
- 1/2 lb ground lamb or beef
- 1 can (14 oz) crushed tomatoes
- 1 medium onion, chopped
- 1 clove garlic, minced
- 1/4 cup red wine
- 2 tbsp tomato paste
- 1/2 tsp cinnamon
- 1/4 cup grated Parmesan cheese
- 2 tbsp olive oil
- For the béchamel: 2 tbsp butter, 2 tbsp flour, 1 1/4 cups milk, nutmeg, salt, and pepper

DIRECTIONS

Sauté the eggplant slices in olive oil until golden, then set aside. In a pan, cook the ground meat with onion and garlic, add red wine, and let it evaporate. Mix in the tomatoes, tomato paste, and cinnamon, cooking until the sauce thickens. Prepare the béchamel by melting butter, blending flour to form a roux, then gradually adding milk until smooth. Season with salt, pepper, and nutmeg. Layer eggplant, meat, and béchamel in a baking dish, finishing with a sprinkle of Parmesan. Bake at 375°F (190°C) for 45 minutes or until golden. Rest before serving.

CALORIES	PROTEIN	FATS	FIBRE
800 KCAL	35G	55G	6G

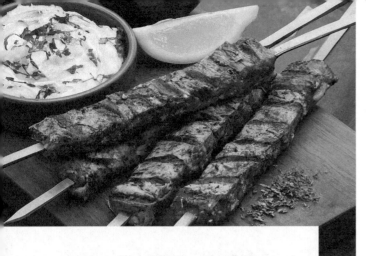

Lamb Souvlaki

(Greece)

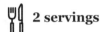 2 servings 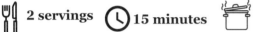 15 minutes 10 minutes

INGREDIENTS

- 1 lb lamb, cubed
- 2 tbsp olive oil
- Juice of 1 lemon
- 2 cloves garlic, minced
- 1 tsp dried oregano
- Salt and black pepper, to taste

DIRECTIONS

Combine lamb with olive oil, lemon juice, garlic, oregano, salt, and pepper in a bowl, ensuring the meat is evenly coated. Cover and marinate in the refrigerator for at least 2 hours or overnight. Preheat the grill or a grill pan over medium-high heat. Thread the marinated lamb onto skewers, spacing the pieces out. Grill, turning occasionally, until well-cooked and charred on all sides, about 10 minutes. Serve hot, optionally, with tzatziki and lemon slices

CALORIES	PROTEIN	FATS	FIBRE
450 KCAL	40G	30G	0G

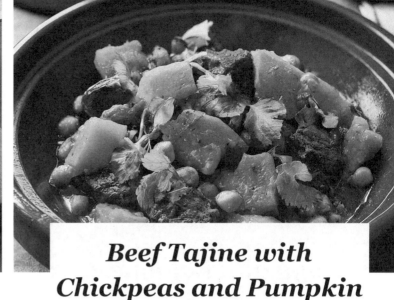

Beef Tajine with Chickpeas and Pumpkin

(Morocco)

 2 servings 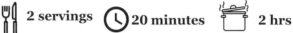 20 minutes 2 hrs

INGREDIENTS

- 1 lb beef, cut into pieces
- 1 cup chickpeas, soaked and drained
- 2 cups pumpkin, cubed
- 1 large onion, chopped
- 2 cloves garlic, minced
- 1 tsp cumin powder
- 1 tsp coriander powder
- 1/2 tsp cinnamon powder
- 2 tbsp olive oil
- 3 cups beef broth
- Salt and black pepper, to taste

DIRECTIONS

In a tajine or heavy pot, heat olive oil over medium heat. Add onion and garlic, sautéing until soft. Mix in beef, chickpeas, pumpkin, cumin, coriander, cinnamon, salt, and pepper. Pour in beef broth to cover the ingredients. Bring to a boil, then reduce heat, cover, and simmer gently for about 2 hours until the beef is tender and the pumpkin easily breaks apart. Adjust seasoning and serve hot directly from the tajine.

CALORIES	PROTEIN	FATS	FIBRE
560 KCAL	48G	24G	6G

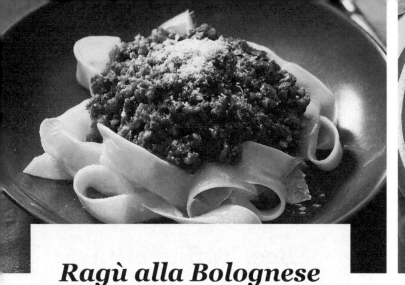

Ragù alla Bolognese

(Italy)

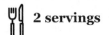 2 servings 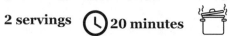 20 minutes   2 hrs

INGREDIENTS

- 1/2 lb ground beef
- 1/4 lb ground pork
- 1 medium carrot, finely chopped
- 1 celery stalk, finely chopped
- 1 medium onion, finely chopped
- 2 cloves garlic, minced
- 1 cup tomato passata
- 1/2 cup red wine
- 1/2 cup whole milk
- 2 tbsp extra virgin olive oil
- Salt and black pepper, to taste
- 1 bay leaf

DIRECTIONS

Heat olive oil in a large pot and sauté onion, carrot, celery, and garlic until soft. Add the ground meats, breaking them apart with a spoon, and cook until browned. Deglaze with red wine, then add the tomato passata, milk, bay leaf, salt, and pepper. Stir well, bring to a simmer, then lower the heat to the minimum, cover, and cook gently for at least 2 hours, stirring occasionally. Add warm water if needed to adjust the consistency. Serve over fresh egg pasta, preferably tagliatelle, and finish with grated Parmigiano Reggiano.

CALORIES 650 KCAL	PROTEIN 35G	FATS 47G	FIBRE 2G

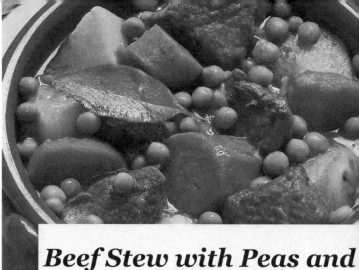

Beef Stew with Peas and Carrots

(Spain)

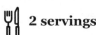 2 servings 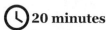 20 minutes 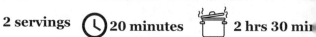 2 hrs 30 min

INGREDIENTS

- 1 lb veal, cubed
- 2 medium potatoes, cubed
- 1 large onion, chopped
- 2 carrots, sliced
- 1/2 cup frozen peas
- 3 cloves garlic, minced
- 1 bay leaf
- 1/2 cup white wine
- 2 cups beef broth
- 2 tbsp extra virgin olive oil
- Salt and black pepper, to taste

DIRECTIONS

In a large pot, heat the oil and brown the veal cubes on all sides. Add onion and garlic and sauté until translucent. Pour in white wine and allow the alcohol to evaporate. Add carrots, potatoes, peas, bay leaf, salt, and pepper. Cover with beef broth and bring to a boil. Reduce heat, cover, and simmer gently for about 2 hours and 30 minutes until the meat is tender and the vegetables are cooked. Season with salt and pepper before serving hot.

CALORIES 720 KCAL	PROTEIN 48G	FATS 35G	FIBRE 5G

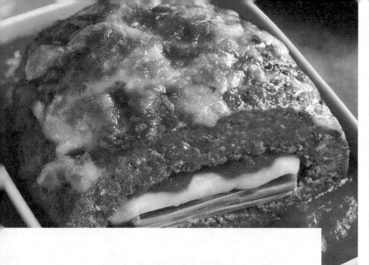

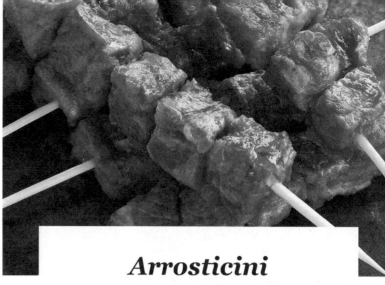

Stuffed Meatloaf

(Italy)

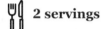 2 servings 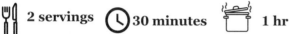 30 minutes 1 hr

INGREDIENTS

- 1 lb ground beef
- 2 slices stale bread, crumbled
- 1/4 cup milk
- 1 large egg
- 1/4 cup grated Parmesan cheese
- 2 cloves garlic, minced
- Salt and black pepper, to taste
- 2 tbsp fresh parsley, chopped
- 4 slices cooked ham
- 1/2 cup mozzarella cheese, cubed
- 1 cup tomato sauce

DIRECTIONS

Begin by soaking the stale bread in milk. Mix the ground beef with the egg, squeezed bread, Parmesan, garlic, parsley, salt, and pepper in a large bowl until well combined. Spread the meat mixture on a piece of parchment paper, forming a rectangle. Evenly distribute the ham slices and mozzarella cubes over the meat, leaving a margin around the edges. Gently roll the meatloaf using the parchment paper and seal the ends. Transfer the meatloaf to a baking dish, top with tomato sauce, and bake in a preheated oven at 375°F (190°C) for about 1 hour. Allow to rest for a few minutes before slicing and serving.

Arrosticini

(Italy)

2 servings 15 minutes 10 minutes

INGREDIENTS

- 1 lb sheep meat, cubed
- Coarse salt and fresh ground black pepper, to taste
- Olive oil for brushing

DIRECTIONS

Thread the cubed sheep meat onto wooden or metal skewers, leaving a small space between each piece for even cooking. Heat a grill or grill pan over medium-high heat. Lightly brush the arrosticini with olive oil and season with coarse salt and black pepper. Grill the skewers, turning frequently, until the meat is golden and cooked to your liking, about 10 minutes. Serve the arrosticini hot, optionally accompanied by slices of bread and a fresh salad.

CALORIES 720 KCAL	PROTEIN 52G	FATS 48G	FIBRE 2G

CALORIES 590 KCAL	PROTEIN 44G	FATS 44G	FIBRE 2G

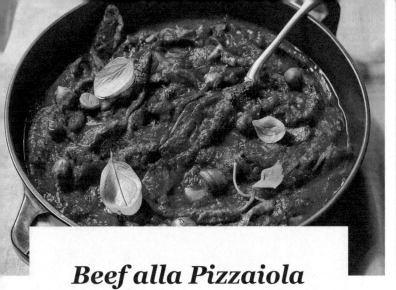

Beef alla Pizzaiola

(Italy)

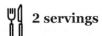 2 servings   10 minutes 20 minutes

INGREDIENTS

- 2 beef steaks, about 1/2 lb each
- 1 can (14 oz) peeled tomatoes
- 2 garlic cloves, thinly sliced
- 2 tbsp extra virgin olive oil
- 1 tsp dried oregano
- Salt and fresh ground black pepper, to taste
- A few fresh basil leaves

DIRECTIONS

Heat the olive oil in a medium skillet over medium heat and sauté the garlic until lightly golden. Add the peeled tomatoes, crushing them with a spoon. Season with oregano, salt, and pepper, and cook the sauce for about 10 minutes until it thickens. Meanwhile, season the steaks with salt and pepper. Add them to the skillet, covering them with the sauce. Cover and cook for about 10 minutes per side, depending on the thickness of the steaks and the desired doneness. Serve the steaks hot, topped with tomato sauce, and garnished with fresh basil leaves.

CALORIES 520 KCAL	PROTEIN 46G	FATS 34G	FIBRE 2G

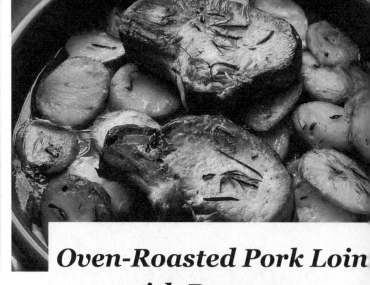

Oven-Roasted Pork Loin with Potatoes

(Spain)

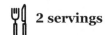 2 servings   15 minutes 1 hr

INGREDIENTS

- 1 lb pork loin
- 4 medium potatoes, cut into wedges
- 4 whole garlic cloves
- 1 sprig of fresh rosemary
- 2 tbsp extra virgin olive oil
- Salt and fresh ground black pepper, to taste
- 1/2 cup white wine

DIRECTIONS

Preheat the oven to 375°F (190°C). Season the pork loin with salt and pepper and place it in a roasting pan. Surround the meat with potato wedges, whole garlic cloves, and rosemary. Drizzle everything with olive oil and pour the white wine into the pan. Roast for about 1 hour until the meat is cooked and the potatoes are golden and tender. Halfway through, turn the potatoes to ensure even browning. Let the meat rest for a few minutes before slicing. Serve the sliced loin with the roasted potatoes and cooked garlic, using the pan juices as a sauce.

CALORIES 640 KCAL	PROTEIN 52G	FATS 26G	FIBRE 5G

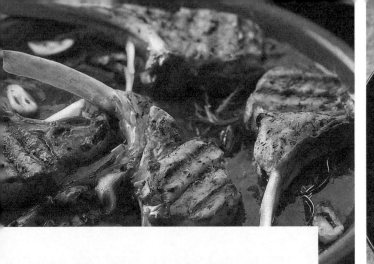

Grilled Lamb Chops

(Spain)

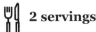 2 servings 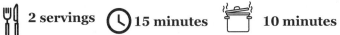 15 minutes   10 minutes

INGREDIENTS

- 4 lamb chops
- 2 tbsp extra virgin olive oil
- 2 garlic cloves, minced
- 1 tsp fresh rosemary, chopped
- 1 tsp fresh thyme, chopped
- Coarse salt and fresh ground black pepper, to taste

DIRECTIONS

Marinate the lamb chops with olive oil, garlic, rosemary, thyme, salt, and pepper, ensuring the meat is well coated. Refrigerate for at least 2 hours, preferably overnight. Preheat the grill to medium-high heat. Remove the lamb from the marinade and grill for 4-5 minutes on each side or until the desired doneness is reached. Let the meat rest for a few minutes before serving to allow the juices to redistribute.

CALORIES 380 KCAL	PROTEIN 24G	FATS 30G	FIBRE 0G

Saltimbocca alla Romana

(Italy)

2 servings 20 minutes 10 minutes

INGREDIENTS

- 4 thin veal slices
- 4 slices of prosciutto
- 8 fresh sage leaves
- 1/4 cup all-purpose flour
- 2 tbsp butter
- 1/2 cup dry white wine
- Salt and fresh ground black pepper, to taste

DIRECTIONS

Slightly flatten the veal slices, then season with salt and pepper. Place a slice of prosciutto and two sage leaves on each veal slice, securing them with toothpicks if needed. Lightly flour both sides of the meat. In a large skillet, melt the butter over medium heat and cook the veal slices for about 3 minutes per side until golden. Remove the meat from the skillet and keep warm. In the same skillet, add the white wine, scraping up the browned bits to create a sauce. Reduce the sauce by half, then pour it over the saltimbocca before serving.

CALORIES 320 KCAL	PROTEIN 22G	FATS 18G	FIBRE 0G

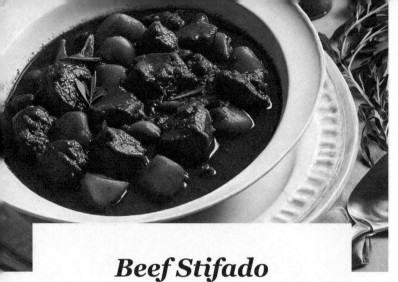

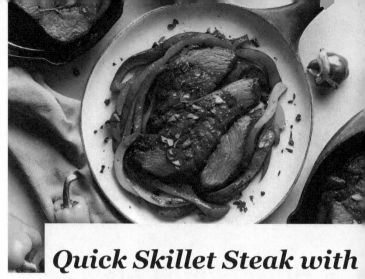

Beef Stifado

(Greece)

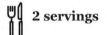 2 servings   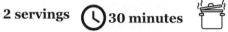 30 minutes   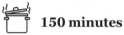 150 minutes

INGREDIENTS

- 1 lb beef, cut into cubes
- 2 tbsp olive oil
- 10-12 small onions, peeled
- 2 garlic cloves, minced
- 1/2 cup red wine
- 2 large tomatoes, peeled and chopped, or 1 can (14 oz) crushed tomatoes
- 1 tbsp red wine vinegar
- 1 bay leaf
- 1 tsp cinnamon powder
- 2 cloves
- Salt and black pepper, to taste

DIRECTIONS

Start by heating the olive oil in a large saucepan over medium-high heat. Add the beef cubes and sauté until they are well browned on all sides, then remove the meat from the saucepan. In the same oil, add the onions and garlic, sautéing until they become translucent. Return the beef to the saucepan along with the red wine, tomatoes, vinegar, bay leaf, cinnamon, cloves, salt, and pepper. Bring to a boil, reduce the heat to low, cover the saucepan, and simmer for about 2 hours and 30 minutes, or until the meat is tender and the sauce has thickened. If necessary, check occasionally and add a bit of water to prevent the sauce from drying out too much. Serve the stifado warm, accompanied by rice or roasted potatoes.

CALORIES	PROTEIN	FATS	FIBRE
600 KCAL	58G	24G	3G

Quick Skillet Steak with Bell Peppers

(Spain)

 4 servings   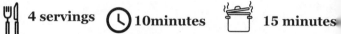 10minutes   15 minutes

INGREDIENTS

- 4 sirloin steaks (about 6 oz each)
- 2 bell peppers (1 red, 1 yellow), sliced
- 2 tablespoons olive oil
- 2 garlic cloves, minced
- 1 teaspoon smoked paprika
- Salt and pepper, to taste
- Fresh parsley, chopped, for garnish

DIRECTIONS

Heat olive oil in a large skillet over medium-high heat. Season steaks with salt, pepper, and smoked paprika. Add steaks to the skillet, cooking for 3-4 minutes on each side for medium-rare or until desired doneness. Remove steaks and set aside. In the same skillet, add sliced bell peppers and minced garlic, sautéing until softened, about 5 minutes. Serve steaks with sautéed bell peppers and a sprinkle of fresh parsley.

CALORIES	PROTEIN	FATS	FIBRE
320 KCAL	25G	22G	2G

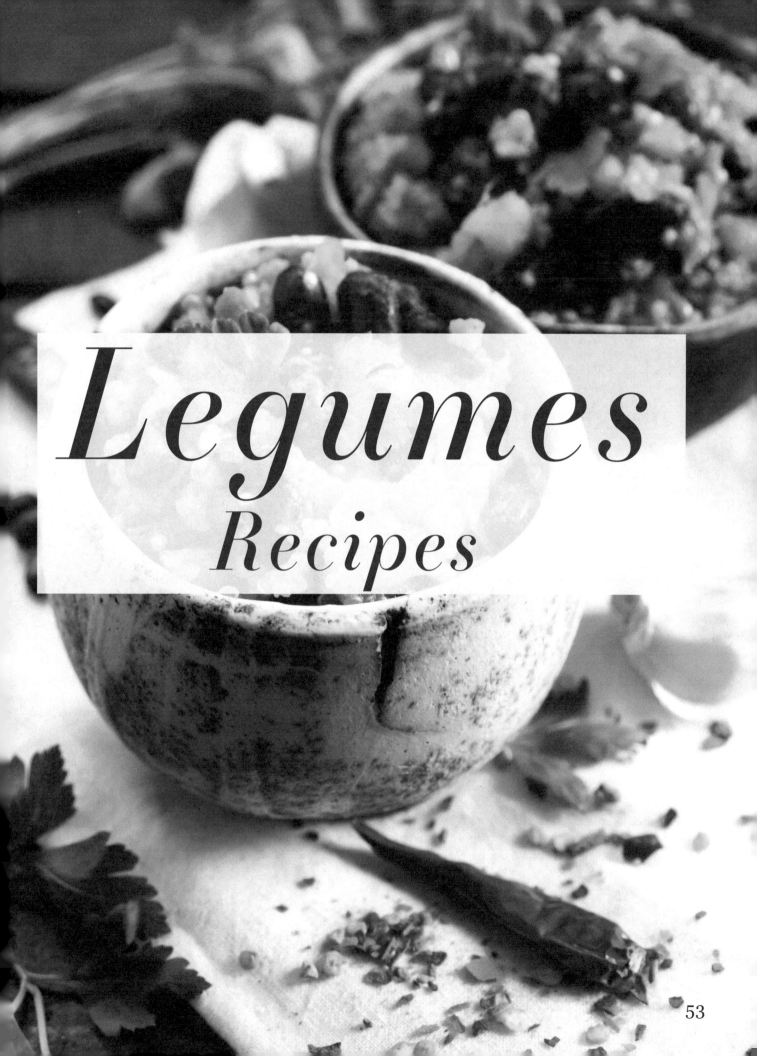

Legumes
Recipes

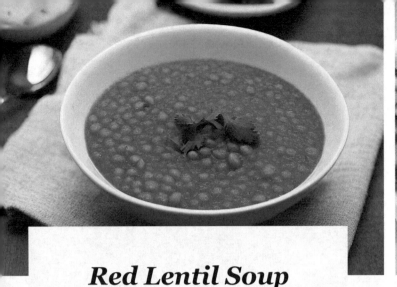

Red Lentil Soup

(Turkey)

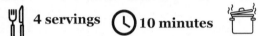 4 servings 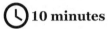 10 minutes 30 minutes

INGREDIENTS

- 1 cup red lentils, rinsed
- 4 cups vegetable broth or water
- 1 medium onion, finely chopped
- 1 carrot, diced
- 2 cloves garlic, minced
- 1 teaspoon paprika
- 1/2 teaspoon ground cumin
- 2 tablespoons extra virgin olive oil
- Salt and black pepper, to taste
- Juice of 1 lemon
- Fresh parsley or cilantro, chopped, for garnish

DIRECTIONS

In a large pot, heat the olive oil over medium heat. Add the onion, carrot, and garlic, sautéing until soft, about 5 minutes. Stir in the red lentils, paprika, and cumin, mixing well. Add the vegetable broth or water and bring to a boil. Reduce heat, cover, and simmer for 25-30 minutes or until the lentils are fully cooked and tender. An immersion blender partially blends the soup, leaving some pieces whole for texture. Season with salt, pepper, and lemon juice. Serve hot, garnished with fresh parsley or cilantro and a drizzle of olive oil.

CALORIES 250 KCAL	PROTEIN 15G	FATS 5G	FIBRE 11G

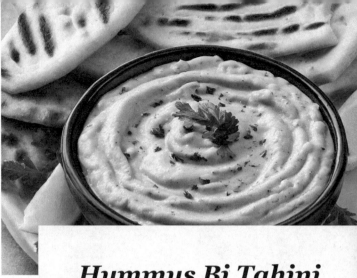

Hummus Bi Tahini

(Middle East)

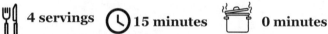 4 servings 15 minutes 0 minutes

INGREDIENTS

- 1 can (15 oz) chickpeas, rinsed and drained
- 1/4 cup tahini (sesame paste)
- 1/4 cup fresh lemon juice
- 1 clove garlic, minced
- 2 tablespoons extra virgin olive oil, plus more for serving
- Salt, to taste
- Paprika or cumin, for garnish
- Pita bread for serving

DIRECTIONS

Combine chickpeas, tahini, lemon juice, garlic, olive oil, and a pinch of salt in a food processor. Blend until smooth and creamy. Add some water or olive oil to reach the desired consistency if the hummus is too thick. Taste and adjust salt as needed. Transfer the hummus to a bowl, create a well in the center with the back of a spoon, and pour a stream of olive oil. Sprinkle with paprika or cumin. Serve with slices of pita bread.

CALORIES 210 KCAL	PROTEIN 7G	FATS 14G	FIBRE 6G

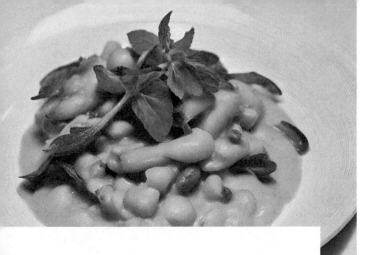

Fava Beans and Chicory

(Italy, Puglia)

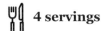 4 servings 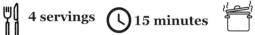 15 minutes   1 hour

INGREDIENTS

- 1 cup dried fava beans, soaked overnight
- 4 cups wild chicory or spinach, cleaned
- 2 cloves garlic, minced
- 4 tablespoons extra virgin olive oil, plus extra for serving
- Salt and black pepper, to taste
- Red chili flakes, optional

DIRECTIONS

Rinse the soaked fava beans and transfer them to a large pot. Cover with fresh water and bring to a boil. Reduce heat and simmer for about 1 hour or until the fava beans are tender. Mash them with a fork or a food mill to obtain a puree. Heat 2 tablespoons of olive oil in a separate pan and sauté the garlic until golden. Add the chicory or spinach, cover, and cook until wilted, about 5-7 minutes. Season with salt, pepper, and chili flakes if used. Serve the fava bean puree warm, topped with the sautéed greens or on the side, drizzled with extra olive oil and an additional sprinkle of pepper.

CALORIES 290 KCAL	PROTEIN 15G	FATS 14G	FIBRE 12G

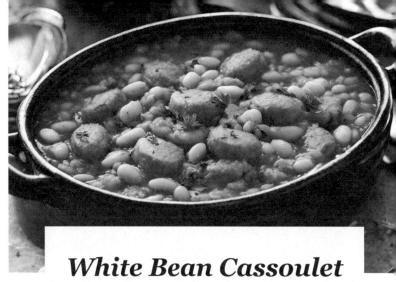

White Bean Cassoulet

(France, South)

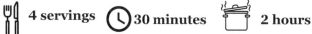 4 servings   30 minutes 2 hours

INGREDIENTS

- 1 cup dry white beans, soaked overnight
- 2 sausages, cut into pieces
- 4 slices of bacon, cut into pieces
- 1 large onion, chopped
- 2 carrots, diced
- 2 cloves garlic, minced
- 1 can (14 oz) diced tomatoes
- 4 cups chicken or vegetable broth
- 1 bouquet garni (thyme, bay leaf, parsley)
- 2 tablespoons breadcrumbs
- 2 tablespoons extra virgin olive oil
- Salt and black pepper, to taste

DIRECTIONS

Rinse the soaked beans and cook them in fresh water for about 1 hour or until tender, then drain. In a large casserole, heat the olive oil and sauté the bacon, sausages, onion, carrots, and garlic until golden. Add the tomatoes, cooked beans, broth, and bouquet garni. Bring to a boil, then reduce heat, partially cover, and simmer for about 1 hour and 30 minutes. If necessary, add more broth to keep the beans covered. Uncover and sprinkle with breadcrumbs in the last 10 minutes of cooking to create a crust. Remove the bouquet garni before serving.

CALORIES 550 KCAL	PROTEIN 35G	FATS 22G	FIBRE 15G

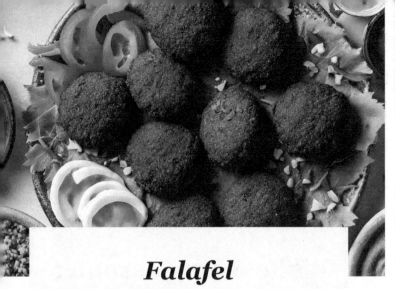
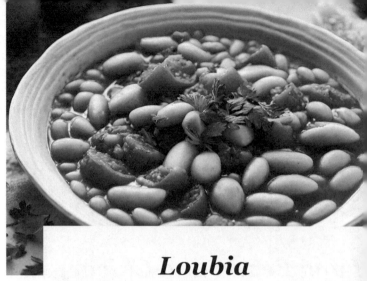

Falafel

(Middle East)

🍴 4 servings   🕐 20 minutes   🍲 10 minutes

INGREDIENTS

- 1 cup dried chickpeas, soaked overnight
- 1 small onion, finely chopped
- 2 cloves garlic, minced
- 1/2 cup fresh parsley, chopped
- 1/2 cup fresh cilantro, chopped
- 1 teaspoon ground cumin
- 1 teaspoon ground coriander
- 1/2 teaspoon chili powder or flakes
- Salt and black pepper, to taste
- Oil for frying

DIRECTIONS

Drain and rinse the soaked chickpeas. Combine chickpeas, onion, garlic, parsley, cilantro, cumin, coriander, chili, salt, and pepper in a food processor. Blend until smooth but still slightly chunky for texture. If necessary, add a little water to help bind the mixture. Let the mixture rest for 15 minutes. Heat oil in a deep fryer or pan to 350°F (175°C). Shape the falafel mixture into balls or patties and fry in the hot oil until golden and crispy, about 5 minutes. Drain on paper towels. Serve the falafel hot with fresh salad, tahini, or hummus, wrapped in pita bread if desired.

CALORIES 300 KCAL	PROTEIN 13G	FATS 15G	FIBRE 9G

Loubia

(Morocco)

🍴 4 servings   🕐 20 minutes   🍲 90 minutes

INGREDIENTS

- 1 cup dry white beans, soaked overnight
- 2 tablespoons extra virgin olive oil
- 1 large onion, chopped
- 2 cloves garlic, minced
- 1 red bell pepper, diced
- 1 can (14 oz) diced tomatoes
- 2 teaspoons ground cumin
- 1 teaspoon paprika
- 1/2 teaspoon chili powder (optional)
- 4 cups water or vegetable broth
- Salt and black pepper, to taste
- Fresh cilantro for garnish

DIRECTIONS

Drain and rinse the soaked white beans. In a large pot, heat the olive oil over medium heat. Add the onion and garlic, sautéing until translucent. Incorporate the red bell pepper and cook for another 5 minutes. Add the tomatoes, cumin, paprika, chili powder (if using), white beans, and water or broth. Bring to a boil, then reduce the heat, cover, and simmer for about 1 hour and 30 minutes or until the beans are tender. Season with salt and pepper. Serve the loubia hot, garnished with chopped fresh cilantro.

CALORIES 250 KCAL	PROTEIN 14G	FATS 5G	FIBRE 12G

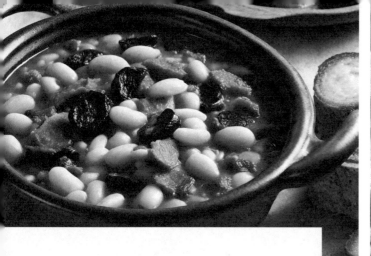

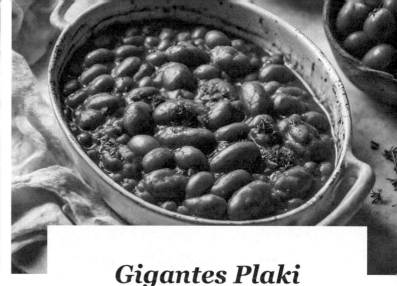

Fabada Asturiana

(Spain, Asturias)

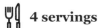 4 servings 30 minutes 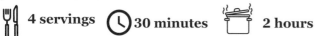 2 hours

INGREDIENTS

- 1 cup dry white beans, soaked overnight
- 2 chorizos, sliced
- 2 morcillas (blood sausage), sliced
- 4 slices of ham, diced
- 1 large onion, chopped
- 2 cloves garlic, minced
- 1 red bell pepper, chopped
- 1 bay leaf
- 1 teaspoon sweet paprika
- Salt and black pepper, to taste
- 6 cups of light broth or water

DIRECTIONS

Drain the soaked beans. Combine beans, chorizo, morcilla, ham, onion, garlic, bell pepper, bay leaf, paprika, salt, and pepper in a large pot and cover with broth or water. Bring to a boil, then lower the heat and simmer gently for about 2 hours or until the beans are very tender and the stew has thickened. Taste and adjust seasoning as needed. Serve the fabada hot, accompanied by crusty bread.

CALORIES 550 KCAL	PROTEIN 35G	FATS 25G	FIBRE 15G

Gigantes Plaki

(Greece)

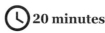 4 servings 20 minutes 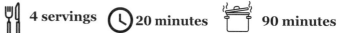 90 minutes

INGREDIENTS

- 1 cup giant beans, soaked overnight
- 1 large onion, chopped
- 2 cloves garlic, minced
- 1 can (14 oz) crushed tomatoes
- 1/4 cup extra virgin olive oil
- 1 teaspoon dried oregano
- 2 bay leaves
- Salt and black pepper, to taste
- Water as needed

DIRECTIONS

Drain and rinse the soaked beans. Cook them in fresh water until almost tender, about 50-60 minutes, then drain again. In a skillet, sauté onion and garlic in olive oil until soft. Add the tomatoes, oregano, bay leaves, salt, and pepper. Combine beans with the tomato sauce and transfer to a baking dish. Cover with aluminum foil and bake in a preheated oven at 350°F (175°C) for about 1 hour and 30 minutes, adding water if necessary to keep the beans moist. Serve the Gigantes place warm or at room temperature.

CALORIES 400 KCAL	PROTEIN 20G	FATS 10G	FIBRE 18G

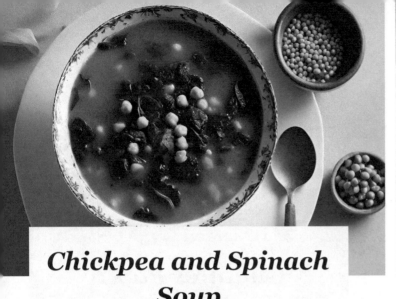

Chickpea and Spinach Soup
(Spain, Andalusia)

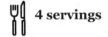 4 servings 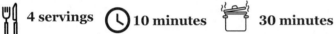 10 minutes 30 minutes

INGREDIENTS

- 1 cup dried chickpeas, soaked overnight, or 2 cups canned chickpeas, rinsed and drained
- 4 cups fresh spinach, washed and roughly chopped
- 1 large onion, chopped
- 2 cloves garlic, minced
- 1 teaspoon sweet paprika
- 1/2 teaspoon ground cumin
- 4 cups vegetable broth or water
- 2 tablespoons extra virgin olive oil
- Salt and black pepper, to taste
- Lemon slices, for serving

DIRECTIONS

In a large pot, heat the olive oil over medium heat. Add the onion and garlic, sautéing until translucent. Incorporate the paprika and cumin, stirring well. Add the chickpeas and vegetable broth. Bring to a boil, then reduce heat and simmer for about 20 minutes or until the chickpeas are tender. Add the spinach and cook for another 5-10 minutes. Season with salt and pepper. Serve the soup hot, accompanied by lemon slices on the side.

CALORIES	PROTEIN	FATS	FIBRE
320 KCAL	18G	10G	12G

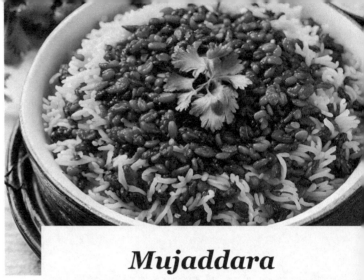

Mujaddara
(Lebanon)

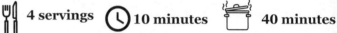 4 servings 10 minutes 40 minutes

INGREDIENTS

- 1 cup green lentils, rinsed
- 1/2 cup basmati rice, rinsed
- 3 large onions, thinly sliced
- 1/2 teaspoon ground cumin
- 3 tablespoons extra virgin olive oil
- Salt and black pepper, to taste
- Water as needed
- Greek yogurt or salad for serving

DIRECTIONS

In a medium pot, cook the lentils in boiling water for about 20 minutes or until tender but not mushy, then drain. Add the rice, cooked lentils, cumin, and enough water to cover by a couple of inches in the same pot. Bring to a boil, reduce heat, cover, and simmer for 20 minutes or until the rice is cooked. Meanwhile, heat the olive oil in a skillet and add the onions, cooking over medium-low heat until caramelized, about 15-20 minutes. Stir regularly to prevent burning. Season the mujaddara with salt and pepper. Serve warm, topped with caramelized onions and Greek yogurt or fresh salad.

CALORIES	PROTEIN	FATS	FIBRE
360 KCAL	14G	10G	15G

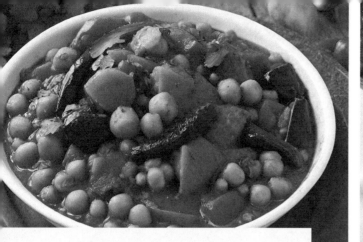

Chickpea and Vegetable Tagine

(Algeria)

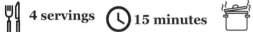 4 servings 15 minutes 1 hour

INGREDIENTS

- 1 cup dried chickpeas, soaked overnight, or 2 cups canned chickpeas, rinsed and drained
- 1 large zucchini, diced
- 2 carrots, diced
- 1 large onion, chopped
- 2 cloves garlic, minced
- 1 can (14 oz) crushed tomatoes
- 1 teaspoon ground cumin
- 1 teaspoon ground coriander
- 1/2 teaspoon chili powder or flakes
- 1/2 teaspoon turmeric
- 4 cups vegetable broth
- 2 tablespoons extra virgin olive oil
- Salt and black pepper, to taste
- Fresh coriander, for garnish

DIRECTIONS

Heat the olive oil over medium heat in a tagine or a heavy pot. Add onion and garlic, sautéing until soft. Stir in cumin, coriander, chili, and turmeric, cooking for a minute until aromatic. Add chickpeas, carrots, zucchini, tomatoes, and vegetable broth. Bring to a boil, then reduce heat, cover, and simmer gently for about 1 hour until vegetables and chickpeas are tender. Season with salt and pepper to taste. Serve the tagine hot, garnished with fresh coriander.

CALORIES 330 KCAL	PROTEIN 15G	FATS 7G	FIBRE 14G

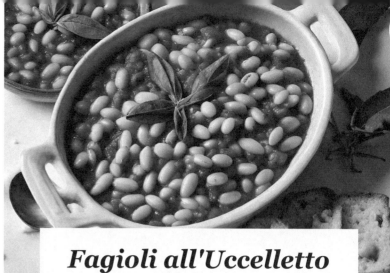

Fagioli all'Uccelletto

(Italy, Tuscany)

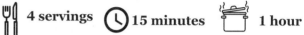 4 servings 15 minutes 1 hour

INGREDIENTS

- 1 cup cannellini beans, dry, soaked overnight
- 2 cloves garlic, minced
- 1 sprig of fresh sage
- 1 red chili pepper, chopped (optional)
- 1 can (14 oz) diced tomatoes
- 3 tablespoons extra virgin olive oil
- Salt and black pepper, to taste

DIRECTIONS

Drain the soaked beans and cook them in a pot of fresh water for about 30 minutes or until tender. Drain again. In a large skillet, heat the olive oil and sauté the garlic, sage, and chili pepper until the garlic turns golden. Add the tomatoes and cook over medium heat for 10 minutes. Incorporate the beans, season with salt and pepper, and simmer for 30 minutes until the sauce thickens. Serve warm as a side dish or main course.

CALORIES 280 KCAL	PROTEIN 14G	FATS 10G	FIBRE 12G

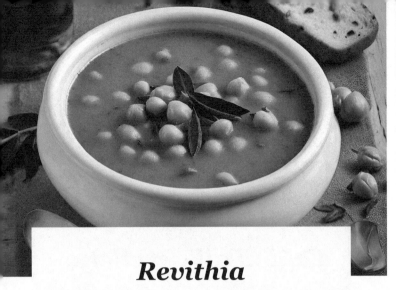

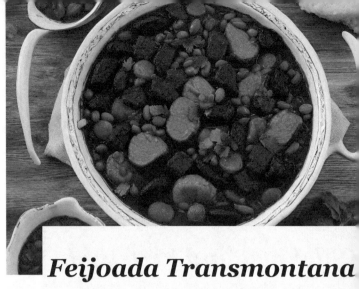

Revithia

(Greece, Cyclades)

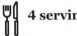 4 servings   10 minutes 🍲 2 hours

INGREDIENTS

- 1 cup dried chickpeas, soaked overnight
- 1 large onion, chopped
- 2 cloves garlic, minced
- 1 bay leaf
- 1/4 cup extra virgin olive oil
- Salt and black pepper, to taste
- Water as needed
- Lemon slices and fresh coriander or parsley for serving

DIRECTIONS

Drain and rinse the soaked chickpeas. Please place them in a large pot with enough fresh water to cover them generously. Add the onion, garlic, and bay leaf, and boil. Reduce heat, partially cover, and simmer for about 2 hours or until the chickpeas are very tender. During cooking, skim off any foam and add hot water to keep the chickpeas covered. Remove the bay leaf, season with salt and pepper, and mix in the olive oil. Serve hot with lemon slices and fresh coriander or parsley.

CALORIES	PROTEIN	FATS	FIBRE
350 KCAL	18G	14G	10G

Feijoada Transmontana

(Portugal)

🍴 4 servings 🕐 30 minutes 🍲 3 hours

INGREDIENTS

- 1 cup black beans, dried, soaked overnight
- 4 oz chorizo, sliced
- 4 oz bacon, cubed
- 1 blood sausage (morcilla), sliced (optional)
- 1 large onion, chopped
- 2 cloves garlic, minced
- 2 bay leaves
- 1/2 teaspoon smoked paprika
- Salt and black pepper, to taste
- Water as needed
- Olive oil, for sautéing

DIRECTIONS

Drain the soaked beans. In a large pot, sauté the onion, garlic, bacon, and chorizo in some olive oil. Once the onion is translucent and the bacon has rendered some fat, add the beans, bay leaves, paprika, salt, pepper, and enough water to cover. Bring to a boil, then reduce heat and simmer covered for about 3 hours, until the beans are tender and the stew has reached a rich consistency. If using, add the blood sausage in the last 30 minutes of cooking. Serve the feijoada hot.

CALORIES	PROTEIN	FATS	FIBRE
600 KCAL	35G	25G	15G

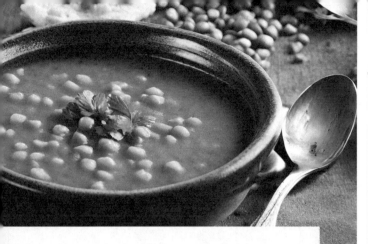
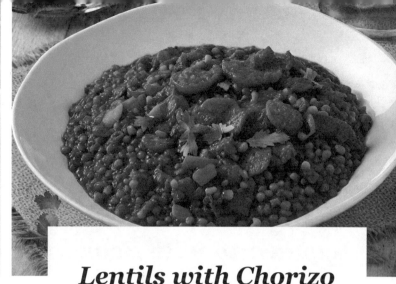

Moroccan Split Pea Soup

(Morocco)

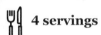 4 servings 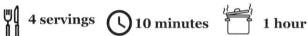 10 minutes 1 hour

INGREDIENTS

- 2 cups dried split peas or dried broad beans, soaked overnight
- 6 cups water
- 2 cloves garlic, minced
- 1 teaspoon ground cumin
- 1/2 teaspoon paprika
- 1/4 teaspoon chili powder (optional)
- 1/4 cup extra virgin olive oil
- Salt, to taste
- Additional olive oil and cumin for serving

DIRECTIONS

Drain and rinse the split peas or broad beans. Place them in a large pot with the water, garlic, cumin, paprika, chili (if using), and a pinch of salt. Bring to a boil, then reduce heat and simmer covered for about 1 hour and 30 minutes or until very tender and beginning to fall apart. Remove from heat and blend with an immersion blender until smooth. Adjust salt and stir in the olive oil. Serve hot with an extra olive oil drizzle and a cumin sprinkle.

CALORIES	PROTEIN	FATS	FIBRE
290 KCAL	18G	10G	14G

Lentils with Chorizo

(Spain)

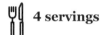 4 servings 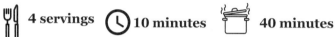 10 minutes 40 minutes

INGREDIENTS

- 1 cup green lentils, rinsed
- 4 cups chicken or vegetable broth
- 2 cloves garlic, minced
- 1 medium onion, chopped
- 2 chorizo sausages, sliced
- 1 red bell pepper, diced
- 1 teaspoon smoked paprika
- 2 tablespoons extra virgin olive oil
- Salt and black pepper, to taste
- Fresh parsley for garnish

DIRECTIONS

In a large pot, heat the olive oil over medium heat. Add the onion and garlic, sautéing until they become transparent. Stir in the chorizo and cook for a few minutes until it releases its oil. Add the bell pepper and paprika and mix well. Add the lentils and broth, boil, then reduce heat and simmer for 30-40 minutes or until the lentils are tender. Season with salt and pepper to taste. Serve hot, garnished with chopped fresh parsley.

CALORIES	PROTEIN	FATS	FIBRE
380 KCAL	22G	14G	18G

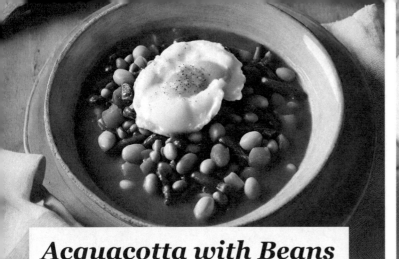

Acquacotta with Beans and Vegetables

(Italy)

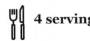 4 servings 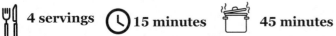 15 minutes 45 minutes

INGREDIENTS

- 1 cup cannellini beans, pre-cooked or canned
- 1 large onion, chopped
- 2 carrots, sliced
- 2 celery stalks, chopped
- 2 cloves garlic, minced
- 1 can (14 oz) crushed tomatoes
- 4 cups vegetable broth
- 4 eggs (optional to serve a poached egg in each dish)
- 4 slices of rustic bread, toasted
- 2 tablespoons extra virgin olive oil
- Salt and black pepper, to taste
- Fresh parsley, chopped, for garnish

DIRECTIONS

In a large pot, heat the olive oil over medium heat. Add the onion, carrots, celery, and garlic, sautéing until soft. Stir in the tomatoes and cook for another 5 minutes. Add the beans and vegetable broth. Bring to a boil, reduce heat, and simmer for 30 minutes. If using eggs, make small wells in the broth with a spoon and crack an egg into each. Cover the pot and cook for about 4 minutes until the egg whites are set but the yolks are still soft. Serve the acquacotta hot over slices of toasted bread garnished with fresh parsley.

CALORIES 280 KCAL	PROTEIN 12G	FATS 7G	FIBRE 10G

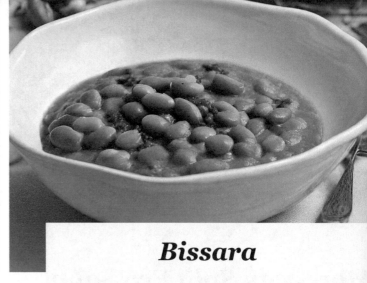

Bissara

(Morocco)

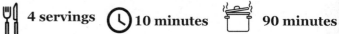 4 servings 10 minutes 90 minutes

INGREDIENTS

- 2 cups dried split peas or broad beans, soaked overnight
- 6 cups water
- 2 cloves garlic, minced
- 1 teaspoon ground cumin
- 1/2 teaspoon paprika
- 1/4 teaspoon chili powder (optional)
- 1/4 cup extra virgin olive oil
- Salt, to taste
- More olive oil and cumin for serving

DIRECTIONS

Drain and rinse the split peas or broad beans. In a large pot, combine them with water, garlic, cumin, paprika, chili (if using), and a pinch of salt. Bring to a boil, then reduce heat and simmer covered for about 1 hour and 30 minutes or until very tender and beginning to disintegrate. Remove from heat and blend with an immersion blender until smooth. Adjust seasoning and mix in the olive oil. Serve hot, drizzled with more olive oil, and sprinkled with cumin.

CALORIES 290 KCAL	PROTEIN 18G	FATS 10G	FIBRE 14G

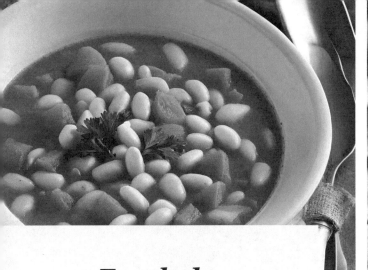
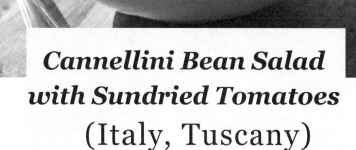

Fasolada

(Greece)

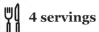 4 servings 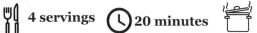 20 minutes 1 hour

INGREDIENTS

- 1 cup dried white beans, soaked overnight
- 1 large onion, chopped
- 2 carrots, sliced
- 2 celery stalks, chopped
- 1 can (14 oz) crushed tomatoes
- 1/4 cup extra virgin olive oil
- 6 cups water or vegetable broth
- 1 bay leaf
- Salt and black pepper, to taste
- Fresh parsley, chopped, for serving

DIRECTIONS

Drain and rinse the soaked beans. In a large pot, heat the olive oil over medium heat. Add the onion, carrots, and celery, sautéing until soft. Stir in the tomatoes and cook for another 5 minutes. Add the beans, water or vegetable broth, and bay leaf. Bring to a boil, then reduce heat and simmer covered for about 1 hour until the beans are tender. Adjust seasoning with salt and pepper. Serve the fasolada hot, garnished with chopped fresh parsley.

Cannellini Bean Salad with Sundried Tomatoes

(Italy, Tuscany)

 4 servings 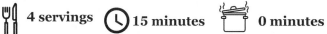 15 minutes 0 minutes

INGREDIENTS

- 2 cans (15 oz each) of cannellini beans, rinsed and drained
- 1/2 cup sundried tomatoes, chopped
- 1/4 cup red onion, finely chopped
- 1/4 cup fresh basil leaves, chopped
- 2 tablespoons capers, rinsed
- 1/4 cup extra virgin olive oil
- 2 tablespoons balsamic vinegar
- Salt and pepper, to taste
- Arugula or mixed greens for serving

DIRECTIONS

Combine a large bowl of cannellini beans, sundried tomatoes, red onion, basil, and capers. Whisk together the olive oil and balsamic vinegar in a small bowl, then pour over the bean mixture. Gently toss to ensure all ingredients are well coated. Season with salt and pepper according to taste. Let the salad sit for about 10 minutes to allow flavors to meld. Serve over a bed of fresh arugula or mixed greens.

CALORIES 320 KCAL	PROTEIN 19G	FATS 7G	FIBRE 16G

CALORIES 290 KCAL	PROTEIN 10G	FATS 14G	FIBRE 8G

Whole Grains
Recipes

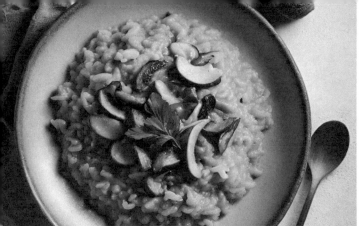

Whole Grain Mushroom Risotto

(Italy)

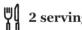 2 servings 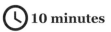 10 minutes 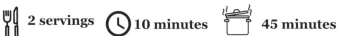 45 minutes

INGREDIENTS

- 1 cup of whole-grain rice
- 2 cups of vegetable broth
- 1/2 cup dried porcini mushrooms, rehydrated and chopped
- 1 small onion, chopped
- 2 cloves of garlic, chopped
- 1/2 cup of white wine
- 2 tablespoons of extra virgin olive oil
- Salt and black pepper, to taste
- Grated Parmigiano Reggiano, to serve
- Fresh parsley, chopped, for garnish

DIRECTIONS

Start by sautéing the onion and garlic in olive oil in a large saucepan over medium heat until they become translucent. Add the whole grain rice, toasting it lightly for a few minutes. Pour in the white wine and let it evaporate. Add the porcini mushrooms and the hot vegetable broth, one ladle at a time, allowing the rice to absorb the liquid before adding more. Continue for about 45 minutes or until the rice is cooked but still al dente. Season with salt and pepper. Serve hot, topped with grated Parmigiano Reggiano and a sprinkle of fresh parsley.

CALORIES 350 KCAL	PROTEIN 12G	FATS 8G	FIBRE 6G

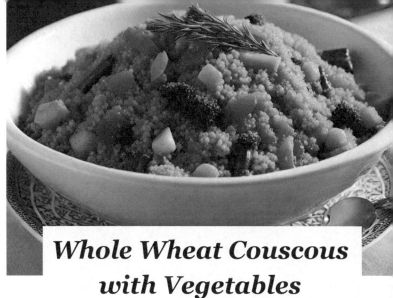

Whole Wheat Couscous with Vegetables

(Morocco)

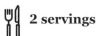 2 servings 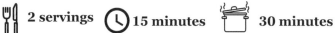 15 minutes 30 minutes

INGREDIENTS

- 1 cup of whole wheat couscous
- 2 cups of vegetable broth
- 1 zucchini, cubed
- 1 carrot, cubed
- 1 red bell pepper, cubed
- 1 onion, chopped
- 2 cloves of garlic, chopped
- 1 teaspoon of ground cumin
- 1/2 teaspoon of ground coriander
- 1/2 teaspoon of paprika
- 2 tablespoons of extra virgin olive oil
- Salt and black pepper, to taste
- Fresh cilantro for garnish

DIRECTIONS

Cook the whole wheat couscous in boiling vegetable broth according to the package instructions. Meanwhile, in a large skillet, heat the olive oil and sauté the onion and garlic until they become translucent. Add the zucchini, carrot, bell pepper, and spices, cooking until the vegetables are tender but still crisp. Mix the cooked couscous with the vegetables in the skillet, stirring well. Serve hot, garnished with chopped fresh cilantro.

CALORIES 320 KCAL	PROTEIN 9G	FATS 7G	FIBRE 8G

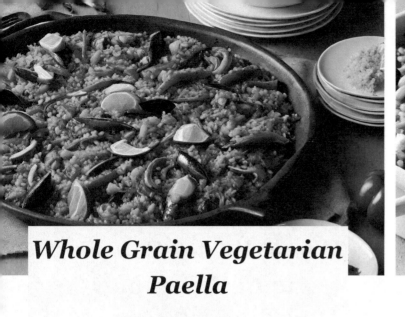

Whole Grain Vegetarian Paella

(Spain)

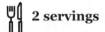 2 servings   🕐 20 minutes   🍲 40 minutes

INGREDIENTS

- 1 cup of whole-grain rice
- 2 1/2 cups of vegetable broth
- 1/2 cup of fresh or frozen peas
- 1 red bell pepper, sliced
- 1 zucchini, cubed
- 1 onion, chopped
- 2 cloves of garlic, chopped
- 1/2 teaspoon of saffron
- 2 tablespoons of extra virgin olive oil
- Salt and black pepper, to taste
- Lemon wedges to serve

DIRECTIONS

Heat the olive oil and sauté the onion and garlic until transparent in a large skillet or paella pan. Add the whole-grain rice and toast it for a few minutes. Incorporate the bell pepper, zucchini, and peas. Add the hot vegetable broth and saffron and mix well. Cook over medium-low heat without stirring until the rice has absorbed the liquid and is cooked for about 40 minutes. Serve the paella hot with lemon wedges on the side.

CALORIES	PROTEIN	FATS	FIBRE
380 KCAL	10G	7G	9G

Baked Barley with Feta and Olives

(Greece)

🍴 2 servings   🕐 15 minutes   🍲 25 minutes

INGREDIENTS

- 1 cup of barley
- 2 cups of vegetable broth
- 1/2 cup of Kalamata olives, pitted and halved
- 1/2 cup of cherry tomatoes, halved
- 1/2 cup of feta cheese, crumbled
- 2 tablespoons of extra virgin olive oil
- 1 teaspoon of dried oregano
- Salt and black pepper, to taste

DIRECTIONS

Preheat the oven to 375°F (190°C). Mix the barley and vegetable broth in a baking dish. Add the olives, cherry tomatoes, olive oil, oregano, salt, and pepper, stirring well to combine the ingredients. Cover the dish with aluminum foil and bake in the oven for about 25 minutes until the barley is tender and has absorbed most of the liquid. Remove the foil, add the crumbled feta on top of the barley, and bake for another 5 minutes until the feta starts to brown slightly. Serve hot.

CALORIES	PROTEIN	FATS	FIBRE
400 KCAL	14G	14G	8G

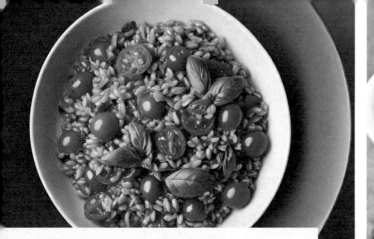

Farro with Cherry Tomatoes and Basil

(Italy)

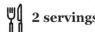 2 servings  10 minutes 30 minutes

INGREDIENTS

- 1 cup of farro, rinsed
- 2 cups of water or vegetable broth
- 1 cup of cherry tomatoes, halved
- 1/4 cup of fresh basil, chopped
- 2 tablespoons of extra virgin olive oil
- Salt and black pepper, to taste
- Parmigiano Reggiano shavings, to serve (optional)

DIRECTIONS

Bring the water or vegetable broth to a boil in a medium pot. Add the farro and reduce the heat to medium-low. Cover and simmer until the farro is tender and has absorbed most of the liquid, about 30 minutes. Drain any excess liquid and transfer the farro to a large bowl. Add the halved cherry tomatoes, chopped fresh basil, olive oil, salt, and pepper. Gently stir to combine. If desired, serve the farro warm or at room temperature, topped with Parmigiano Reggiano shavings.

CALORIES 300 KCAL	PROTEIN 10G	FATS 6G	FIBRE 7G

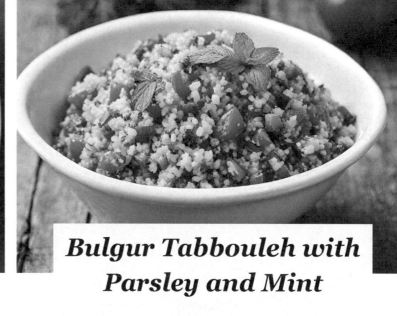

Bulgur Tabbouleh with Parsley and Mint

(Cyprus)

 2 servings 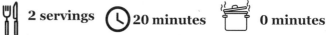 20 minutes 0 minutes

INGREDIENTS

- 1/2 cup of bulgur
- 1 cup of boiling water
- 1 large bunch of parsley, finely chopped
- 1/4 cup of fresh mint, finely chopped
- 2 medium tomatoes, diced
- 1/4 cup of red onion, finely chopped
- 2 tablespoons of extra virgin olive oil
- Juice of 1 large lemon
- Salt and black pepper, to taste

DIRECTIONS

Pour the bulgur into a large bowl and add the boiling water. Cover and let stand for about 10-15 minutes, or until the bulgur has absorbed all the water and is soft. Once ready, fluff the bulgur with a fork to separate the grains. Add parsley, mint, tomatoes, red onion, olive oil, and lemon juice to the bulgur. Season with salt and pepper to your taste. Stir well until all ingredients are thoroughly combined. Let the tabbouleh rest in the refrigerator for at least 1 hour before serving, allowing the flavors to meld. Serve chilled as a refreshing side dish or as part of a larger meal.

CALORIES 220 KCAL	PROTEIN 6G	FATS 10G	FIBRE 8G

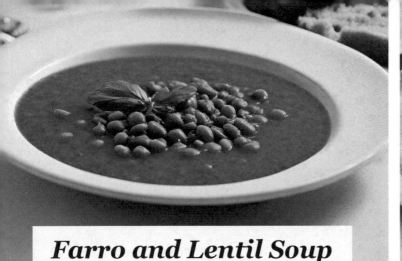

Farro and Lentil Soup

(Italy)

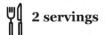 2 servings   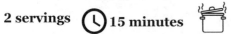 15 minutes   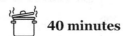 40 minutes

INGREDIENTS

- 1/2 cup of farro
- 1/2 cup of green lentils
- 1 medium carrot, diced
- 1 stalk of celery, diced
- 1 small onion, chopped
- 2 cloves of garlic, chopped
- 4 cups of vegetable broth
- 2 tablespoons of extra virgin olive oil
- Salt and black pepper, to taste
- Grated Parmigiano Reggiano for serving, optional

DIRECTIONS

In a large pot, heat the olive oil over medium heat. Add the onion, celery, carrot, and garlic, sautéing until they soften. Incorporate the farro and lentils, stirring for a couple of minutes to lightly toast them. Add the vegetable broth and bring to a boil. Reduce the heat, cover the pot, and simmer for 30-40 minutes, or until both farro and lentils are tender. Adjust the seasoning with salt and pepper to your taste. Serve the soup hot, sprinkled with grated Parmigiano Reggiano, if desired.

CALORIES 380 KCAL	PROTEIN 15G	FATS 7G	FIBRE 10G

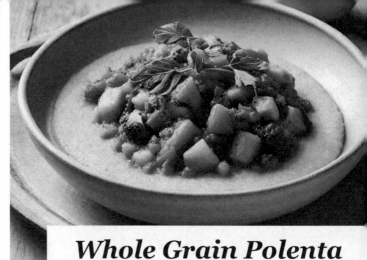

Whole Grain Polenta with Vegetable Ragù

(Italy)

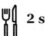 2 servings   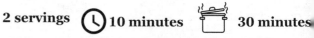 10 minutes   30 minutes

INGREDIENTS

- 1 cup of whole-grain polenta
- 4 cups of water
- 1 zucchini, cubed
- 1 red bell pepper, cubed
- 1 carrot, cubed
- 1 onion, chopped
- 2 cloves of garlic, chopped
- 1 can (14 oz) of diced tomatoes
- 2 tablespoons of extra virgin olive oil
- Salt and black pepper, to taste
- Fresh basil for garnish

DIRECTIONS

Bring water to a boil in a large pot and slowly pour in the polenta, stirring constantly to avoid lumps. Reduce the heat to low and continue cooking, stirring frequently, until the polenta has thickened, about 20-30 minutes. Meanwhile, in another skillet, heat the olive oil over medium heat and sauté the onion and garlic until they become transparent. Add zucchini, bell pepper, and carrot, and cook until the vegetables soften. Incorporate the diced tomatoes, salt, and pepper, and simmer until a thick ragù is achieved about 10 minutes. Serve the hot polenta, topped with the vegetable ragù and garnished with fresh basil leaves.

CALORIES 320 KCAL	PROTEIN 7G	FATS 9G	FIBRE 6G

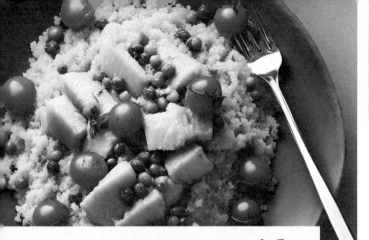

Farro Couscous with Swordfish

(Sicily, Italy)

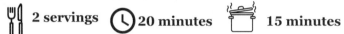 2 servings | 20 minutes | 15 minutes

INGREDIENTS

- 1 cup farro couscous
- 2 swordfish steaks, about 6 oz each
- 1/2 cup cherry tomatoes, halved
- 1/4 cup capers, rinsed
- 2 tablespoons extra virgin olive oil, plus extra for drizzling
- 1 lemon, juiced
- Salt and black pepper, to taste
- Fresh basil for garnish

DIRECTIONS

Cook the farro couscous according to package instructions and keep warm. Meanwhile, heat a skillet over medium-high heat and add 2 tablespoons of olive oil. Season the swordfish steaks with salt and pepper, then cook in the hot skillet for 3-4 minutes on each side or until golden and cooked to the desired doneness. Remove the fish from the skillet and keep warm. Add the cherry tomatoes and capers in the same skillet, cooking for a few minutes until the tomatoes break down. Return the fish to the skillet, add lemon juice, and cook for another minute, gently mixing. Serve the farro couscous on plates, top with the swordfish, tomatoes, and capers, drizzle with olive oil and garnish with fresh basil leaves.

CALORIES 450 KCAL	PROTEIN 35G	FATS 12G	FIBRE 8G

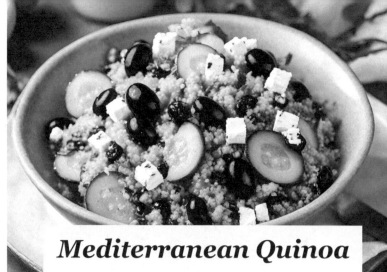

Mediterranean Quinoa

(Greece)

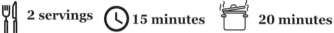 2 servings | 15 minutes | 20 minutes

INGREDIENTS

- 1 cup quinoa
- 2 cups water or vegetable broth
- 1/2 cup cucumbers, diced
- 1/2 cup cherry tomatoes, halved
- 1/4 cup Kalamata olives, pitted and halved
- 1/4 cup feta cheese, crumbled
- 2 tablespoons extra virgin olive oil
- 1 lemon, juiced
- Salt and black pepper, to taste
- Fresh parsley, chopped, for garnish

DIRECTIONS

Rinse the quinoa well under cold running water. In a medium pot, bring the water or vegetable broth to a boil, add the quinoa, reduce the heat to low, cover, and cook until all the water is absorbed, about 15 minutes. Let the quinoa cool slightly, then transfer it to a large bowl. Add the cucumbers, cherry tomatoes, olives, feta, olive oil, lemon juice, salt, and pepper. Gently mix to combine all the ingredients. Garnish with chopped fresh parsley before serving.

CALORIES 340 KCAL	PROTEIN 12G	FATS 9G	FIBRE 7G

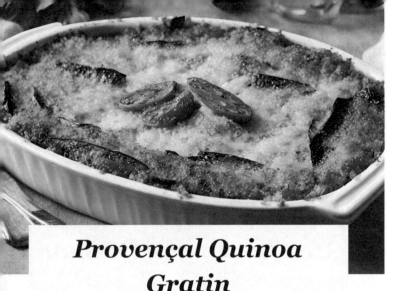

Provençal Quinoa Gratin

(France)

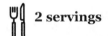 2 servings 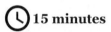 15 minutes 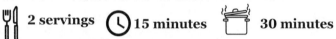 30 minutes

INGREDIENTS

- 1 cup quinoa, rinsed
- 2 cups vegetable broth
- 1 zucchini, thinly sliced
- 1 small eggplant, thinly sliced
- 2 tomatoes, thinly sliced
- 1/4 cup Parmigiano Reggiano, grated
- 2 tablespoons extra virgin olive oil
- 1 clove garlic, minced
- Salt and black pepper, to taste
- Herbes de Provence, to taste

DIRECTIONS

Preheat the oven to 375°F (190°C). Cook the quinoa in vegetable broth according to package instructions until soft and all the liquid has been absorbed. In a baking dish, alternate layers of cooked quinoa with zucchini, eggplant, and tomatoes, sprinkling each layer with salt, pepper, Herbes de Provence, minced garlic, and a drizzle of olive oil. Finish the top layer with grated Parmigiano Reggiano. Bake in the oven for about 20-30 minutes, until the surface is golden, and vegetables are tender. Serve hot as a main dish or side.

CALORIES 420 KCAL	PROTEIN 16G	FATS 14G	FIBRE 8G

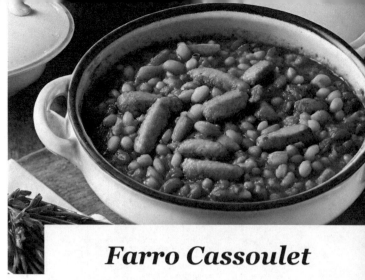

Farro Cassoulet

(France)

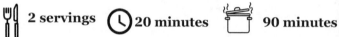 2 servings   20 minutes 90 minutes

INGREDIENTS

- 1 cup farro, soaked overnight and drained
- 4 cups vegetable broth
- 2 vegetarian sausages, sliced
- 1 carrot, diced
- 1 onion, chopped
- 2 cloves of garlic, chopped
- 1 can (14 oz) diced tomatoes
- 1 bay leaf
- 1 sprig of thyme
- Salt and black pepper, to taste
- Breadcrumbs, optional
- 2 tablespoons extra virgin olive oil

DIRECTIONS

In a large casserole, heat the olive oil over medium heat. Add the onion, garlic, and carrot, sautéing until soft. Add the vegetarian sausages and cook for a few minutes. Incorporate the farro, diced tomatoes, bay leaf, thyme, salt, and pepper. Pour in the vegetable broth and bring to a boil. Reduce the heat, cover, and simmer for about 1 hour and 30 minutes, or until the farro is tender. If you desire a crispy crust, transfer the cassoulet to a baking dish, sprinkle with breadcrumbs, and broil under the grill for 5-10 minutes until golden. Serve hot.

CALORIES 480 KCAL	PROTEIN 18G	FATS 12G	FIBRE 10G

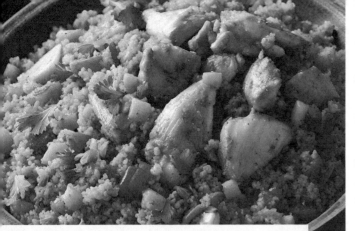

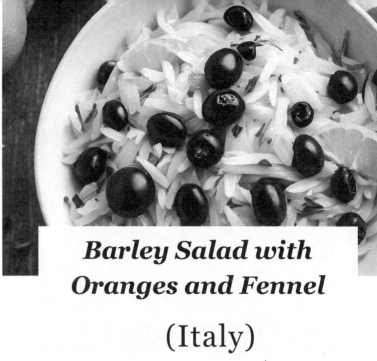

ulgur with Chicken and Vegetables

(Morocco)

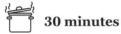

🍴 2 servings 🕐 20 minutes 🍲 30 minutes

INGREDIENTS

1 cup bulgur
2 cups chicken broth
2 chicken breasts, cut into bite-sized pieces
1 zucchini, cubed
1 red bell pepper, cubed
1 small onion, chopped
2 cloves of garlic, chopped
1 teaspoon turmeric
1 teaspoon cumin
2 tablespoons extra virgin olive oil
Salt and black pepper, to taste
Fresh cilantro, chopped, for garnish

DIRECTIONS

Bring the chicken broth to a boil in a medium pot and add the bulgur. Reduce the heat, cover, and cook until the bulgur has absorbed all the broth, about 15-20 minutes. Meanwhile, heat the olive oil over medium-high heat in a large skillet. Add the chicken seasoned with salt and pepper, and sauté until golden, then set aside. Add the onion, garlic, zucchini, and bell pepper in the same skillet, season with turmeric and cumin, and cook until the vegetables are tender. Mix the chicken back into the skillet, combine with the cooked bulgur, and heat together for a few minutes. Serve hot, garnished with chopped cilantro.

CALORIES 360 KCAL	PROTEIN 24G	FATS 8G	FIBRE 9G

Barley Salad with Oranges and Fennel

(Italy)

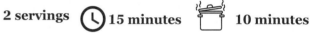

🍴 2 servings 🕐 15 minutes 🍲 10 minutes

INGREDIENTS

- 1 cup barley
- 2 oranges, peeled and cut into segments
- 1 fennel bulb, thinly sliced
- 1/4 cup black olives, pitted
- 2 tablespoons extra virgin olive oil
- 1 lemon, juiced
- Salt and black pepper, to taste
- Fresh mint leaves, for garnish

DIRECTIONS

Cook the barley in boiling salted water according to package instructions, then drain it and let it cool. Combine the cooled barley with the orange segments, sliced fennel, black olives, olive oil, and lemon juice in a large bowl. Season with salt and pepper to taste. Gently mix to combine all the ingredients. Let the salad rest for at least 10 minutes before serving to allow the flavors to meld. Garnish with fresh mint leaves for a touch of freshness.

CALORIES 320 KCAL	PROTEIN 10G	FATS 7G	FIBRE 6G

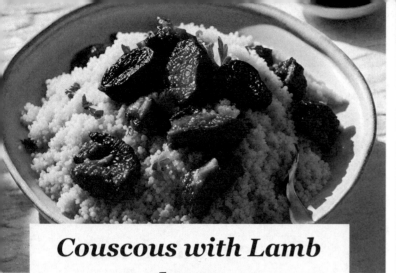

Couscous with Lamb and Prunes

(Morocco)

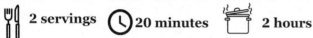 2 servings 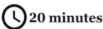 20 minutes 2 hours

INGREDIENTS

- 1/2 lb lamb meat, cut into cubes
- 1 cup whole wheat couscous
- 1/2 cup dried prunes
- 1/4 cup toasted almonds
- 1 medium onion, chopped
- 2 cloves of garlic, chopped
- 1 teaspoon cinnamon powder
- 1/2 teaspoon saffron
- 2 cups meat broth
- 2 tablespoons extra virgin olive oil
- Salt and black pepper, to taste
- Fresh cilantro for garnish

DIRECTIONS

In a large saucepan, heat the olive oil over medium heat. Add the cubed lamb, onion, garlic, and sauté until the meat is well browned. Season with cinnamon, saffron, salt, and pepper. Add the meat broth and bring to a boil. Reduce the heat, cover, and simmer gently for about 1 hour and 30 minutes. Add the dried prunes and cook for 30 minutes until the lamb is tender. Meanwhile, prepare the whole wheat couscous according to the package instructions. Serve the couscous with the lamb and prune mixture on top, garnished with toasted almonds and fresh cilantro.

CALORIES	PROTEIN	FATS	FIBRE
420 KCAL	22G	12G	8G

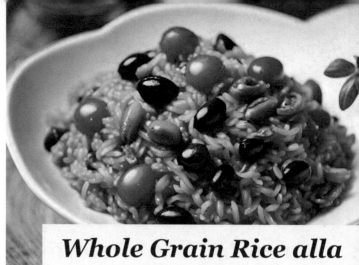

Whole Grain Rice alla Puttanesca

(Italy)

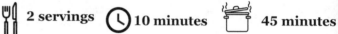 2 servings 10 minutes 45 minutes

INGREDIENTS

- 1 cup whole-grain rice
- 2 cups water or vegetable broth
- 1 can (14 oz) diced tomatoes
- 2 cloves of garlic, chopped
- 1/4 cup black olives, pitted and sliced
- 2 tablespoons capers, rinsed and drained
- 2 anchovy fillets, chopped (optional for a non-vegetarian version)
- 1 red chili pepper, chopped or 1/2 teaspoon chili flakes
- 2 tablespoons extra virgin olive oil
- Salt and black pepper, to taste
- Fresh parsley, chopped, for garnish

DIRECTIONS

Bring the water or vegetable broth to a boil in a medium pot. Add the whole grain rice, reduce the heat, cover it, and cook until it has absorbed all the liquid and becomes tender for about 45 minutes. Meanwhile, heat the olive oil over medium heat in a large skillet. Add the garlic and chili pepper, sautéing for about 1-2 minutes until the garlic is golden. Add the diced tomatoes, olives, capers, and anchovies (if used), and simmer for 15-20 minutes until the sauce thickens. Once the rice is cooked, add it to the skillet with the puttanesca sauce, mixing well to combine. Serve hot, garnished with chopped fresh parsley.

CALORIES	PROTEIN	FATS	FIBRE
380 KCAL	11G	10G	7G

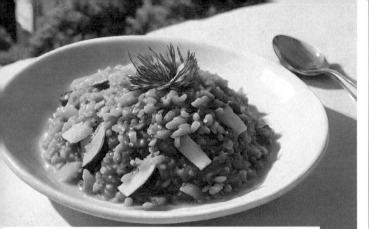

Farro with Artichokes and Pecorino

(Italy)

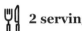 2 servings  15 minutes 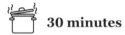 30 minutes

INGREDIENTS

- 1 cup farro
- 2 cups vegetable broth
- 4 fresh artichokes, cleaned and cut into wedges
- 1/2 cup Pecorino Romano, grated
- 2 cloves of garlic, chopped
- 2 tablespoons extra virgin olive oil
- Salt and black pepper, to taste
- Fresh parsley, chopped, for garnish

DIRECTIONS

Cook the farro in a pot with the vegetable broth according to package instructions or until it is tender but still al dente. Meanwhile, heat the olive oil over medium heat in a wide skillet and sauté the garlic for about 1-2 minutes. Add the artichokes and cook, stirring occasionally, until they are golden and tender, about 8-10 minutes. If needed, add a little water to prevent sticking. Once the farro is cooked, drain it and add it to the skillet with the artichokes. Adjust the seasoning with salt and pepper, then mix well to combine all the ingredients. Serve the dish hot, sprinkling with grated Pecorino Romano and garnished with chopped fresh parsley.

CALORIES 350 KCAL	PROTEIN 15G	FATS 9G	FIBRE 8G

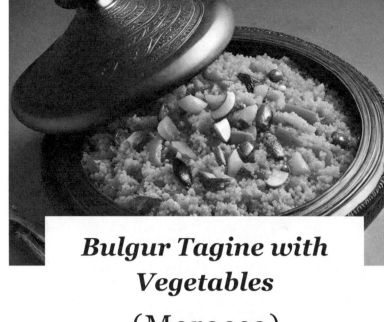

Bulgur Tagine with Vegetables

(Morocco)

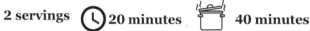 2 servings   20 minutes 40 minutes

INGREDIENTS

- 1 cup bulgur
- 2 cups vegetable broth
- 1 zucchini, cubed
- 1 carrot, cubed
- 1 red bell pepper, cubed
- 1 onion, chopped
- 2 cloves of garlic, chopped
- 1 teaspoon ground cumin
- 1 teaspoon ground coriander
- 1/2 teaspoon paprika
- 1/2 teaspoon turmeric
- 1/4 teaspoon cinnamon
- 1/4 cup cooked chickpeas
- Extra virgin olive oil
- Salt and black pepper, to taste
- Fresh cilantro and lemon slices for garnish

DIRECTIONS

Heat some olive oil over medium heat in a tagine or a heavy-bottomed pot. Add onion and garlic, sautéing until they become translucent. Incorporate zucchini, carrot, bell pepper, chickpeas, and spices (cumin, coriander, paprika, turmeric, and cinnamon), cooking for a few minutes until the vegetables soften. Add the bulgur and stir well to ensure it's fully coated with the spices. Pour in the vegetable broth, boil, then reduce the heat to low, cover, and cook until the bulgur has absorbed all the liquid, about 20 minutes. Let it rest covered for 5 minutes, then fluff with a fork. Serve the bulgur tagine hot, garnished with chopped fresh cilantro and lemon slices.

CALORIES 310 KCAL	PROTEIN 9G	FATS 5G	FIBRE 10G

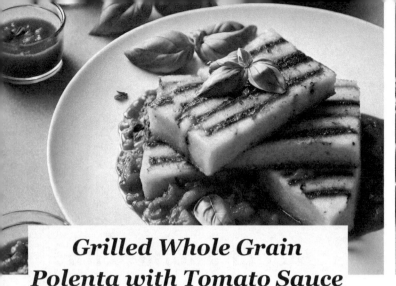

Grilled Whole Grain Polenta with Tomato Sauce

(Italy)

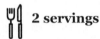 2 servings   10 minutes   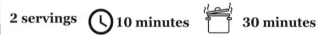 30 minutes

INGREDIENTS

- 1 cup whole-grain polenta
- 4 cups water or vegetable broth
- 1 cup homemade or high-quality tomato sauce
- 2 tablespoons extra virgin olive oil, plus extra for grilling
- Salt and black pepper, to taste
- Fresh basil for garnish

DIRECTIONS

Bring the water or broth to a boil in a large pot. Gradually whisk in the polenta, stirring continuously to prevent lumps. Reduce the heat to low and continue cooking, stirring often, until the polenta thickens and starts to pull away from the sides of the pot, about 25-30 minutes. Pour the polenta onto a tray lined with parchment paper, spreading it into an even layer. Let it cool completely, then cut into squares or rectangles. Heat a grill or grill pan over medium-high heat. Lightly brush the polenta pieces with olive oil and grill them until they have excellent grill marks on both sides. Serve the grilled polenta warm, topped with tomato sauce, and garnished with fresh basil.

CALORIES 290 KCAL	PROTEIN 6G	FATS 7G	FIBRE 5G

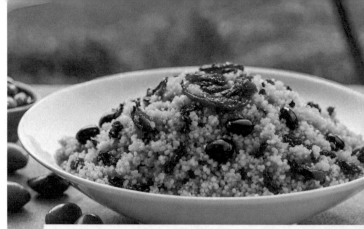

Quinoa with Sun-Dried Tomatoes and Olives

(Italy)

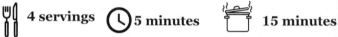 4 servings   5 minutes   15 minutes

INGREDIENTS

- 1 cup quinoa
- 2 cups water
- 1/2 cup sun-dried tomatoes, chopped
- 1/2 cup black olives, pitted and sliced
- 1/4 cup fresh basil, chopped
- 2 tablespoons olive oil
- Salt and pepper to taste

DIRECTIONS

Cook quinoa in water according to package instructions. Once cooked, fluff with a fork and let cool slightly. Stir in sun-dried tomatoes, olives, basil, and olive oil. Season with salt and pepper. Serve either warm or at room temperature.

CALORIES 220 KCAL	PROTEIN 6G	FATS 10G	FIBRE 5G

Pizza bread and Focaccia
Recipes

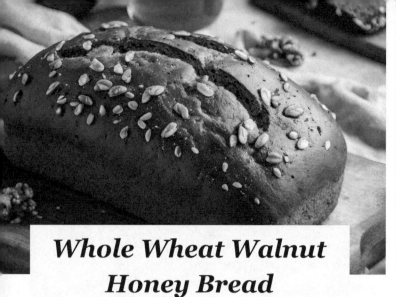

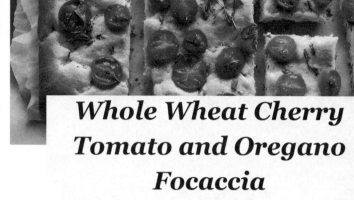

Whole Wheat Walnut Honey Bread

 2 servings   **20 minutes**   **30 minutes**

INGREDIENTS

- 2 cups whole wheat flour
- 1 cup warm water
- 2¼ tsp active dry yeast
- 2 tbsp honey
- ½ cup walnuts, roughly chopped
- 1 tsp salt
- 2 tbsp olive oil

DIRECTIONS

Dissolve yeast in warm water. Mix in flour, honey, salt, yeast, and olive oil. Knead, add walnuts and let rise for 1 hour. Shape, and bake at 375°F for 30 minutes.

Whole Wheat Cherry Tomato and Oregano Focaccia

2 servings    **15 minutes**   **20 minutes**

INGREDIENTS

- 1½ cups whole wheat flour
- ¾ cup warm water
- 1 tsp active dry yeast
- 1 tbsp extra virgin olive oil, plus more for drizzling
- ½ tsp salt
- 1 cup cherry tomatoes, halved
- 1 tbsp fresh oregano, chopped
- Coarse sea salt for sprinkling

DIRECTIONS

Mix yeast, water, flour, oil, and salt. Let rise for 1 hour. Top with tomatoes and oregano, drizzle with oil and sprinkle with salt. Bake at 400°F for 20 minutes.

CALORIES	PROTEIN	FATS	FIBRE
350 KCAL	10G	8G	6G

CALORIES	PROTEIN	FATS	FIBRE
320 KCAL	9G	7G	6G

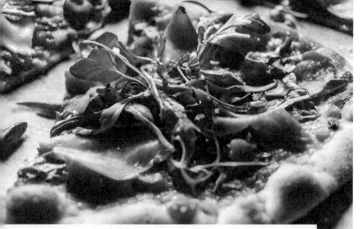

Whole Wheat thin-crust pizza with Arugula and Prosciutto

 2 servings 20 minutes 15 minutes

INGREDIENTS

- 1½ cups whole wheat flour
- ¾ cup water
- 1 tsp active dry yeast
- ½ tsp salt
- 1 tbsp olive oil
- ½ cup tomato sauce
- 1 cup mozzarella cheese, shredded
- ½ cup arugula
- 4 slices prosciutto
- Extra virgin olive oil for drizzling

DIRECTIONS

Make dough with flour, water, yeast, salt, and oil. Rise for 1 hour. Top with sauce and cheese, and bake at 450°F for 10 minutes. Add arugula, prosciutto, drizzle oil.

CALORIES	PROTEIN	FATS	FIBRE
460 KCAL	22G	18G	8G

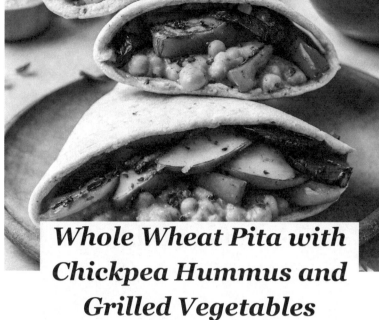

Whole Wheat Pita with Chickpea Hummus and Grilled Vegetables

 2 servings 20 minutes 10 minutes

INGREDIENTS

- 1½ cups whole wheat flour
- ⅔ cup warm water
- 1 tsp active dry yeast
- ½ tsp salt
- 1 tbsp olive oil
- 1 cup homemade or store-bought hummus
- 1 bell pepper, sliced and grilled
- 1 small zucchini, sliced and grilled
- 1 small eggplant, sliced and grilled

DIRECTIONS

Mix flour, yeast, salt, water, and oil. Knead, rise, shape into circles, bake at 475°F for 5 mins. Serve with hummus and vegetables.

CALORIES	PROTEIN	FATS	FIBRE
510 KCAL	19G	20G	14G

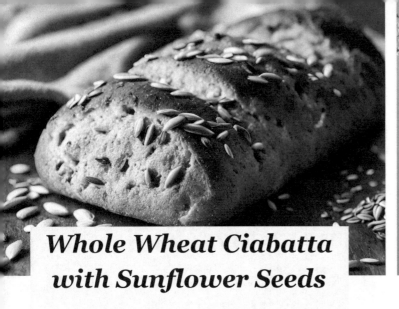
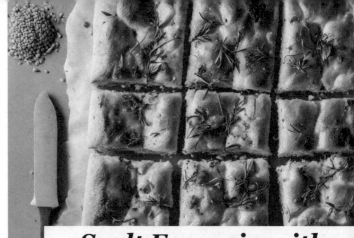

Whole Wheat Ciabatta with Sunflower Seeds

Spelt Focaccia with Caramelized Onion

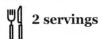 2 servings 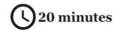 20 minutes 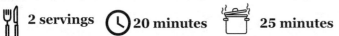 25 minutes

 2 servings 15 minutes 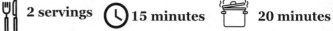 20 minutes

INGREDIENTS

- 1½ cups whole wheat flour
- 1 cup water
- 1 tsp active dry yeast
- ½ tsp salt
- 1 tbsp olive oil
- ¼ cup sunflower seeds

INGREDIENTS

- 1 cup whole wheat flour
- 1 cup spelt flour
- ¾ cup warm water
- 1 tsp active dry yeast
- ½ tsp salt
- 2 tbsp olive oil
- 1 large onion, thinly sliced and caramelized
- Sea salt and rosemary for topping

DIRECTIONS

Mix yeast, water, flour, salt, and oil. Add seeds and rise for 1 hour. Shape and bake at 425°F for 25 mins.

DIRECTIONS

Prepare dough with flour, water, yeast, salt, and oil. Rise for 1 hour. Top with onion, rosemary, and salt. Bake at 400°F for 20 minutes.

CALORIES	PROTEIN	FATS	FIBRE
380 KCAL	12G	10G	8G

CALORIES	PROTEIN	FATS	FIBRE
400 KCAL	13G	9G	10G

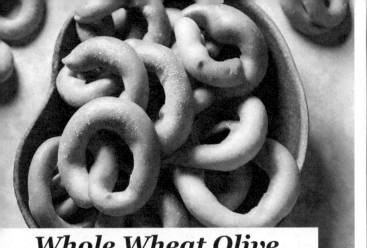
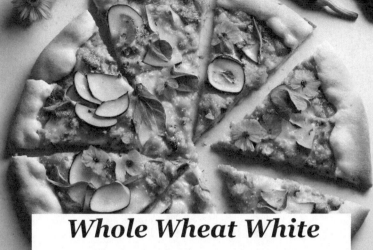

Whole Wheat Olive Taralli

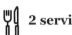 2 servings 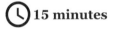 15 minutes  20 minutes

INGREDIENTS

- 2 cups whole wheat flour
- ½ tsp salt
- 2 tbsp olive oil
- ¼ cup chopped black olives
- ½ cup water

DIRECTIONS

Combine flour, salt, olive oil, olives, and water to form dough. Shape into rings, boil for 1 minute and bake at 375°F for 20 mins.

CALORIES 300 KCAL	PROTEIN 8G	FATS 10G	FIBRE 5G

Whole Wheat White Pizza with Zucchini and Squash Blossoms

2 servings 15 minutes 20 minutes

INGREDIENTS

- 1½ cups whole wheat flour
- ¾ cup water
- 1 tsp active dry yeast
- ½ tsp salt
- 2 tbsp olive oil, plus more for drizzling
- ½ cup ricotta cheese
- 1 small zucchini, thinly sliced
- 6 squash blossoms, cleaned and trimmed
- Salt and pepper, to taste

DIRECTIONS

Make dough with flour, water, yeast, salt, and 1 tbsp oil. Let it rise for 1 hour. Stretch onto a baking sheet and top with ricotta, zucchini, and blossoms. Drizzle with oil, season, and bake at 450°F for 20 mins.

CALORIES 450 KCAL	PROTEIN 20G	FATS 15G	FIBRE 10G

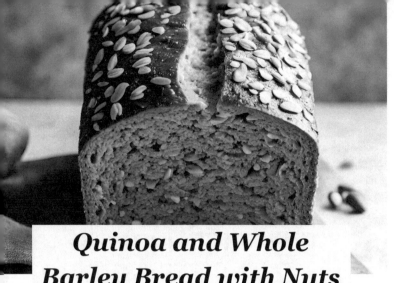

Quinoa and Whole Barley Bread with Nuts

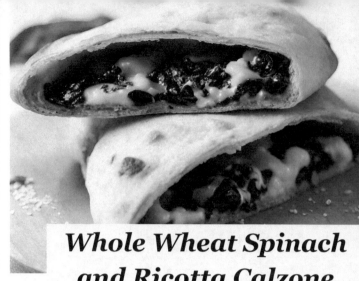

Whole Wheat Spinach and Ricotta Calzone

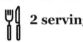 2 servings 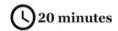 20 minutes 35 minutes

INGREDIENTS

- 1 cup whole wheat flour
- ½ cup cooked quinoa
- ½ cup cooked barley
- 1 tsp active dry yeast
- 1 cup warm water
- ½ tsp salt
- 1 tbsp olive oil
- ¼ cup mixed nuts, chopped

DIRECTIONS

Combine flour, quinoa, barley, yeast, water, salt, and oil. Knead, add nuts and let rise for 1 hour. Shape and bake at 375°F for 35 mins.

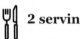 2 servings 20 minutes 25 minutes

INGREDIENTS

- 1½ cups whole wheat flour
- ¾ cup water
- 1 tsp active dry yeast
- ½ tsp salt
- 1 tbsp olive oil
- 1 cup spinach, cooked and drained
- ½ cup ricotta cheese
- ¼ cup mozzarella cheese, shredded
- Salt and pepper, to taste

DIRECTIONS

Prepare dough with flour, water, yeast, salt, and oil. Let rise for 1 hour. Fill half with spinach, ricotta, and mozzarella. Fold, seal, and bake at 425°F for 25 mins.

CALORIES 420 KCAL	PROTEIN 14G	FATS 12G	FIBRE 9G

CALORIES 480 KCAL	PROTEIN 22G	FATS 16G	FIBRE 8G

Dessert
Recipes

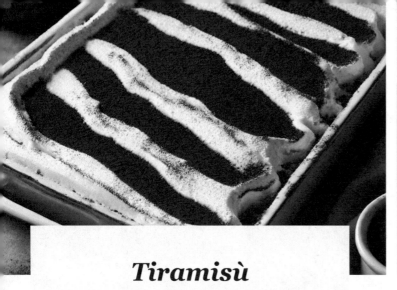

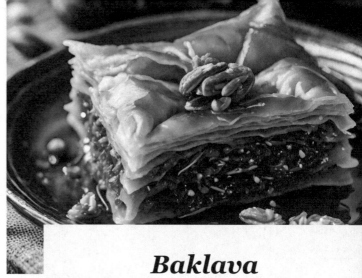

Tiramisù

(Italy)

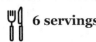 6 servings 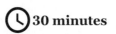 30 minutes 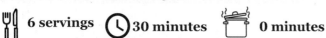 0 minutes

INGREDIENTS

- 3 large eggs, separated
- 3/4 cup granulated sugar
- 1 cup mascarpone cheese
- 1 1/2 cups strong, cold coffee
- 1 package of ladyfingers (about 24 biscuits)
- Cocoa powder, for dusting

DIRECTIONS

Whisk the egg yolks with the sugar until light and fluffy. Incorporate the mascarpone cheese. In another bowl, beat the egg whites until stiff peaks form, and gently fold them into the mascarpone mixture. Dip the ladyfingers in the coffee and lay them out in a layer in a rectangular dish. Cover with half of the mascarpone mixture. Repeat the layers and finish with the cream. Cover and let rest in the refrigerator for at least 4 hours. Before serving, dust with cocoa powder.

CALORIES	PROTEIN	FATS	FIBRE
450KCAL	8G	27G	45G

Baklava

(Turkey/Greece)

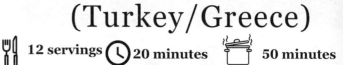 12 servings 20 minutes 50 minutes

INGREDIENTS

- 1 package of phyllo dough, thawed
- 2 cups chopped nuts (walnuts, pistachios, or a combination)
- 1 teaspoon ground cinnamon
- 1 cup melted butter
- 1 cup sugar
- 1 cup water
- 1/2 cup honey
- 1 teaspoon vanilla extract

DIRECTIONS

Mix nuts and cinnamon. Grease a baking dish and layer sheets of phyllo dough, brushing each with melted butter. After half the sheets are laid, evenly distribute the nut mixture. Cover with the remaining sheets, brushing each with butter. Cut into diamonds and bake in a preheated oven at 350°F (175°C) for 50 minutes. Boil water and sugar, add honey and vanilla, and pour the hot syrup over the freshly baked baklava. Allow to absorb and cool completely before serving.

CALORIES	PROTEIN	FATS	FIBRE
330KCAL	4G	20G	35G

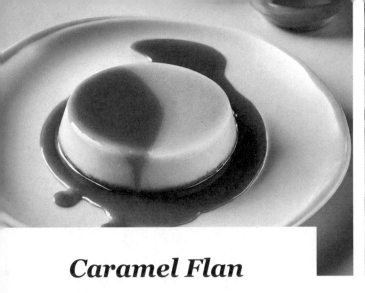
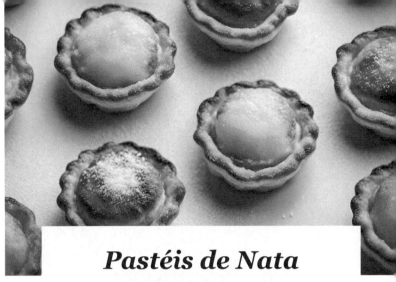

Caramel Flan

(Spain)

6 servings   15 minutes   1 hour

INGREDIENTS

- 3/4 cup sugar, for caramel
- 4 large eggs
- 2 cups whole milk
- 1/2 cup granulated sugar
- 1 teaspoon vanilla extract

DIRECTIONS

Melt 3/4 cup of sugar in a pan until golden caramel forms. Pour it into a flan mold, tilting to cover the bottom and sides. Beat eggs with sugar, milk, and vanilla. Pour into the caramelized mold. Bake in a water bath in the oven at 325°F (165°C) for about 1 hour. Cool and unmold onto a plate before serving.

Pastéis de Nata

(Portugal)

12 servings   30 minutes   20 minutes

INGREDIENTS

- 1 roll of ready-made puff pastry
- 1 cup sugar
- 2 tablespoons cornstarch
- 1 1/2 cups whole milk
- 6 egg yolks
- 1 teaspoon vanilla extract
- Cinnamon and powdered sugar for serving

DIRECTIONS

Roll out the puff pastry and cut circles to line muffin tin cups. Boil milk, sugar, and cornstarch, stirring until it thickens. Remove from heat and slowly incorporate the egg yolks and vanilla. Fill the pastry-lined cups with the mixture and bake in an oven at 400°F (200°C) for 20 minutes, until golden. Dust with cinnamon and powdered sugar before serving.

CALORIES	PROTEIN	FATS	FIBRE
300 KCAL	7G	7G	50G

CALORIES	PROTEIN	FATS	FIBRE
220 KCAL	4G	11G	1G

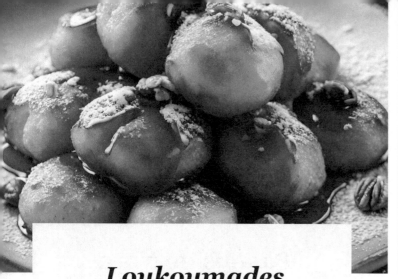

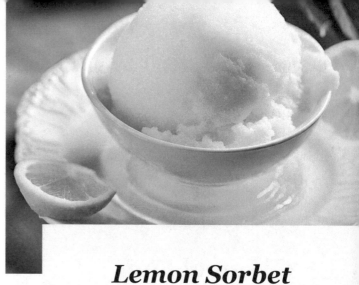

Loukoumades

(Greece)

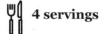 4 servings 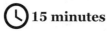 15 minutes 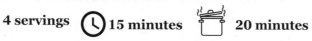 20 minutes

INGREDIENTS

- 1 cup warm water
- 2 teaspoons sugar
- 2 teaspoons active dry yeast
- 2 cups wheat flour
- 1/2 teaspoon salt
- Oil for frying
- Honey for serving
- Ground cinnamon, to taste
- Chopped nuts, optional

DIRECTIONS

Dissolve yeast in warm water with sugar. Add flour and salt, mixing until a smooth dough forms. Cover and let rise in a warm place until doubled in size. Heat oil and fry small portions of dough until golden, then drain and immerse in honey. Sprinkle with cinnamon and nuts, if desired, and serve immediately.

CALORIES 300 KCAL	PROTEIN 5G	FATS 15G	FIBRE 1G

Lemon Sorbet

(Italy)

4 servings   20 minutes/Freezing : 3 hours

INGREDIENTS

- 1 cup fresh lemon juice
- 1 cup water
- 3/4 cup sugar

DIRECTIONS

Boil water and sugar in a saucepan, stirring until the sugar dissolves completely, then let cool. Add the lemon juice to the cooled syrup, mix, and pour into a shallow dish. Freeze until semi-solid, then blend with a mixer to make the sorbet creamy. Freeze again until serving time.

CALORIES 150 KCAL	PROTEIN 0G	FATS 0G	FIBRE 0G

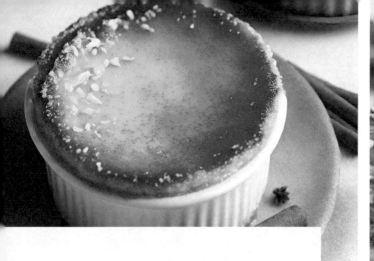

Crème Brûlée

(France)

Prep Time: 15 min | Cook Time: 40 min | Cooling Time: 2 hours | Servings: 4

INGREDIENTS

- 2 cups heavy cream
- 1/2 cup sugar, plus extra for caramelizing
- 5 egg yolks
- 1 teaspoon vanilla extract

DIRECTIONS

Heat the cream with half the sugar and vanilla until it almost boils. Beat the yolks with the remaining sugar until light and fluffy. Slowly add the hot cream to the yolks, stirring constantly. Pour the mixture into ramekins and bake in a water bath at 325°F (165°C) for 40 minutes. Cool, then sprinkle sugar and caramelize with a kitchen torch before serving.

CALORIES 410 KCAL	PROTEIN 5G	FATS 30G	FIBRE 0G

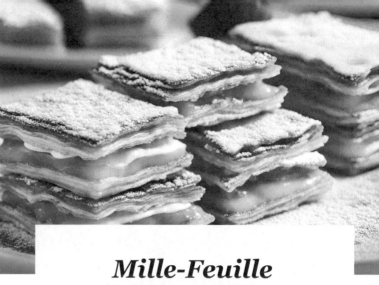

Mille-Feuille

(France)

Prep Time: 30 min | Cook Time: 15 min | Cooling Time: 1 hour | Servings: 4

INGREDIENTS

- 1 package of ready-made puff pastry
- 2 cups of pastry cream
- Powdered sugar, for garnish

DIRECTIONS

Roll out the puff pastry and cut it into equal-sized rectangles. Bake in a preheated oven at 400°F (200°C) until golden. Let cool. Assemble the mille-feuille by alternating layers of puff pastry and pastry cream, ending with a layer of pastry. Dust with powdered sugar before serving.

CALORIES 520 KCAL	PROTEIN 8G	FATS 32G	FIBRE 1G

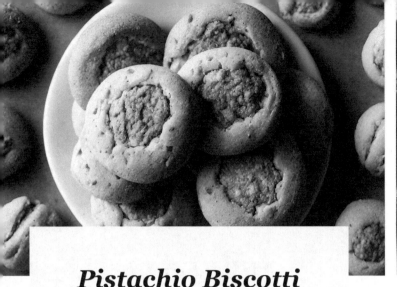

Pistachio Biscotti

(Sicily, Italy)

 20 biscuits 20 minutes 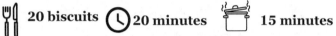 15 minutes

INGREDIENTS

- 1 cup flour
- 1/2 cup sugar
- 1/2 cup chopped pistachios
- 1/4 cup unsalted butter, softened
- 1 large egg
- 1 teaspoon vanilla extract
- A pinch of salt

DIRECTIONS

Mix flour, salt, and pistachios in a bowl. In another bowl, cream together butter and sugar until light. Add the egg and vanilla, then incorporate the dry ingredients to form a dough. Shape into small logs, place on a baking sheet lined with parchment paper, and slightly flatten. Bake in a preheated oven at 350°F (175°C) for about 15 minutes or until golden. Let cool before serving.

CALORIES 100 KCAL	PROTEIN 2G	FATS 5G	FIBRE 1G

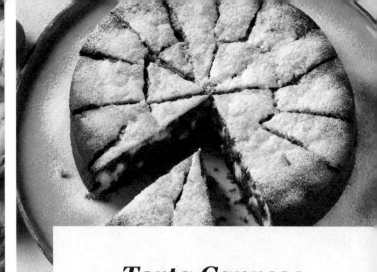

Torta Caprese

(Italy)

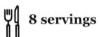 8 servings 15 minutes 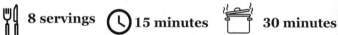 30 minutes

INGREDIENTS

- 1 cup ground almonds
- 3/4 cup sugar
- 1/2 cup unsalted butter, softened
- 4 large eggs
- 1/2 cup cocoa powder
- 1 teaspoon vanilla extract
- Powdered sugar, for garnish

DIRECTIONS

Cream the butter and sugar until light and fluffy. Add eggs one at a time, then vanilla. Mix in ground almonds and cocoa until smooth. Pour into a greased and floured cake pan. Bake at 350°F (175°C) for about 30 minutes. Cool before dusting with powdered sugar.

CALORIES 320 KCAL	PROTEIN 7G	FATS 20G	FIBRE 3G

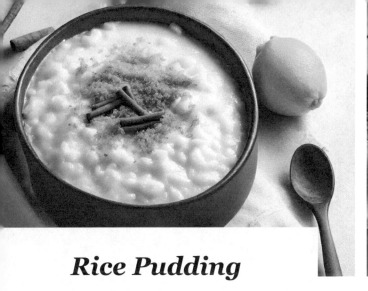

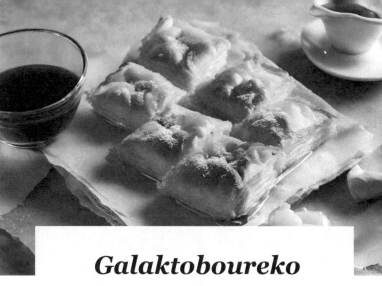

Rice Pudding

(Spain)

🍴 4 servings 🕐 5 minutes 🍲 40 minutes

INGREDIENTS

- 1/2 cup short-grain rice
- 4 cups whole milk
- 1/3 cup sugar
- 1 cinnamon stick
- Zest of 1 lemon
- Ground cinnamon for garnish

DIRECTIONS

Bring the milk to a boil in a saucepan with the cinnamon stick and lemon zest. Add the rice and reduce the heat. Simmer, stirring occasionally, until the rice is tender and the milk is almost completely absorbed, about 40 minutes. Remove from heat, discard the cinnamon stick and lemon zest, stir in the sugar, and mix well. Serve warm or cold, garnished with ground cinnamon.

CALORIES 260 KCAL	PROTEIN 8G	FATS 5G	FIBRE 1G

Galaktoboureko

(Greece)

🍴 6 servings 🕐 30 minutes 🍲 45 minutes

INGREDIENTS

- 1/2 lb phyllo dough
- 1 cup semolina
- 4 cups milk
- 1 cup sugar
- 4 eggs
- 1/4 cup melted butter
- 1 teaspoon vanilla extract
- Zest of 1 lemon
- For the syrup:
- 1 cup sugar
- 1/2 cup water
- Juice of 1/2 lemon

DIRECTIONS

Boil the milk with lemon zest. Add semolina, stirring until thickened. Remove from heat, slightly cool, and add sugar, eggs, and vanilla, mixing well. Grease a baking dish and layer half the phyllo sheets, brushing each with melted butter. Spread the filling and cover with the remaining phyllo, brushing each layer with butter. Bake at 350°F (175°C) for about 45 minutes until golden. For the syrup, cook sugar, water, and lemon juice until thickened and pour over the hot Galaktoboureko. Let cool before serving.

CALORIES 580 KCAL	PROTEIN 12G	FATS 18G	FIBRE 2G

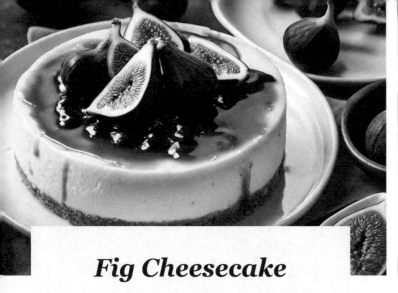
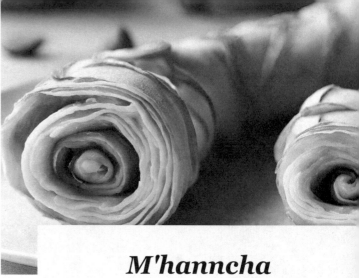

Fig Cheesecake

(Turkey)

Prep Time: 20 min | Cook Time: 1 hour | Cooling Time: 4 hours | Servings: 8

INGREDIENTS

- 1 1/2 cups crushed digestive biscuits
- 1/3 cup melted butter
- 2 cups cream cheese
- 3/4 cup sugar
- 3 eggs
- 1 teaspoon vanilla extract
- 1 cup fresh figs, sliced
- For the fig compote:
- 1 cup fresh or dried figs
- 1/2 cup sugar
- 1/4 cup water

DIRECTIONS

Mix biscuits with melted butter and press into the bottom of a springform pan. Beat cream cheese with sugar, add eggs one at a time, and vanilla. Pour over the crust and top with sliced figs. Bake at 325°F (165°C) for 1 hour. Cool and refrigerate for at least 4 hours. For the compote, cook figs, sugar, and water until a sauce forms. Serve the cheesecake with the fig compote.

CALORIES	PROTEIN	FATS	FIBRE
450 KCAL	7G	27G	2G

M'hanncha

(Morocco)

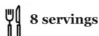 8 servings 25 minutes 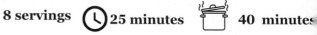 40 minutes

INGREDIENTS

- 1/2 lb phyllo dough
- 2 cups ground almonds
- 1 cup sugar
- 1/2 teaspoon ground cinnamon
- 1/4 teaspoon orange blossom water
- 1/2 cup melted butter
- Powdered sugar, for garnish

DIRECTIONS

Mix the ground almonds with sugar, cinnamon, and orange blossom water. Take a sheet of phyllo, brush it with melted butter, and spread a portion of the almond mixture along one edge. Roll the cigar up to form a long cigar. Coil the cigar into a spiral shape. Repeat with the remaining ingredients. Bake in a preheated oven at 350°F (175°C) until golden. Dust with powdered sugar before serving.

CALORIES	PROTEIN	FATS	FIBRE
320 KCAL	6G	18G	3G

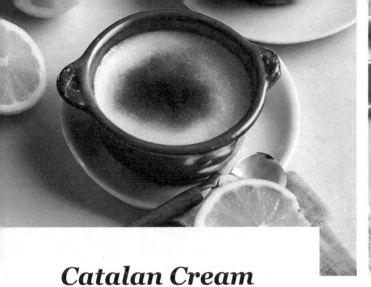

Catalan Cream

(Spain, Catalonia)

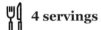 4 servings   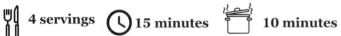 15 minutes   10 minutes

INGREDIENTS

- 2 cups whole milk
- 1 cinnamon stick
- Zest of 1 lemon
- 4 egg yolks
- 1/3 cup sugar
- 2 tablespoons cornstarch
- Sugar, for caramelizing

DIRECTIONS

Heat milk with the cinnamon stick and lemon zest until boiling. In a bowl, beat the yolks with sugar and cornstarch until smooth. Remove the cinnamon and spice from the milk and gradually pour over the yolk mixture, stirring constantly. Return the mixture to heat and cook until it thickens. Pour the cream into bowls, cool, then refrigerate. Before serving, sprinkle with sugar and caramelize with a kitchen torch.

CALORIES 220 KCAL	PROTEIN 6G	FATS 8G	FIBRE 0G

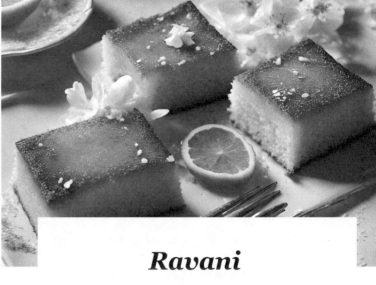

Ravani

(Greece)

8 servings   20 minutes   35 minutes

INGREDIENTS

- 1 cup semolina
- 1/2 cup flour
- 1 teaspoon baking powder
- 4 eggs
- 1 cup sugar
- 1/2 cup Greek yogurt
- 1/2 cup melted butter
- 1 teaspoon vanilla extract
- For the syrup:
- 1 cup water
- 1 cup sugar
- Juice of 1 lemon
- 1 teaspoon rose water (optional)

DIRECTIONS

Mix semolina, flour, and baking powder. Beat eggs with sugar until light in another bowl, then add yogurt, butter, and vanilla. Combine the dry ingredients, pour into a baking dish, and bake at 350°F (175°C) for 35 minutes. For the syrup, cook water, sugar, and lemon juice until thickened, then add rose water. Pour hot syrup over the cake once it's baked. Allow to absorb and cool before serving.

CALORIES 360 KCAL	PROTEIN 5G	FATS 12G	FIBRE 1G

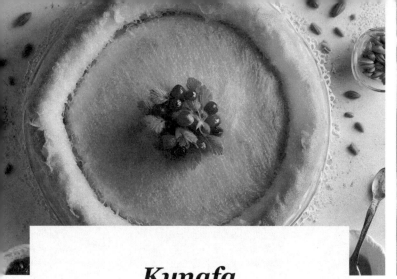

Kunafa

(Middle East)

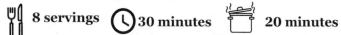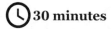

🍴 8 servings 🕐 30 minutes ♨ 20 minutes

INGREDIENTS

- 1/2 lb kuna fa dough or shredded phyllo, finely chopped
- 1/2 cup melted butter
- 2 cups mozzarella cheese or a sweet cheese, grated
- 1/2 cup sugar
- 1/2 cup water
- 1 teaspoon lemon juice
- 1/4 teaspoon rose water or orange blossom water

DIRECTIONS

Combine melted butter with the kunafa dough. Press half of the mixture into a baking dish. Distribute the cheese evenly over the base, then cover with the remaining kunafa mixture. Bake in a preheated oven at 350°F (175°C) for about 20 minutes or until the surface turns golden and crisp. Meanwhile, prepare a syrup by boiling water and sugar until reduced, then add lemon juice and rose or orange blossom water. Pour the hot syrup over the freshly baked kunafa. Let it cool before cutting and serving.

CALORIES 380 KCAL	PROTEIN 10G	FATS 18G	FIBRE 1G

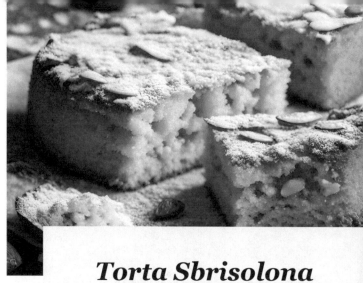

Torta Sbrisolona

(Italy, Lombardy)

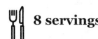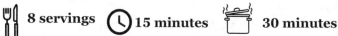

🍴 8 servings 🕐 15 minutes ♨ 30 minutes

INGREDIENTS

- 1 cup almond flour
- 1 cup fine cornmeal
- 1/2 cup sugar
- 1/2 cup whole almonds
- 3/4 cup cold butter, cubed
- 1 egg
- Grated zest of 1 lemon
- A pinch of salt

DIRECTIONS

Mix almond flour, cornmeal, sugar, whole almonds, lemon zest, and salt in a bowl. Add butter and egg, mixing with your fingers until the mixture becomes crumbly. Spread the mixture in a baking pan without pressing down too much. Bake in a preheated oven at 350°F (175°C) until golden and crisp, about 30 minutes. Allow the cake to cool completely before breaking it into irregular pieces to serve.

CALORIES 400 KCAL	PROTEIN 8G	FATS 27G	FIBRE 3G

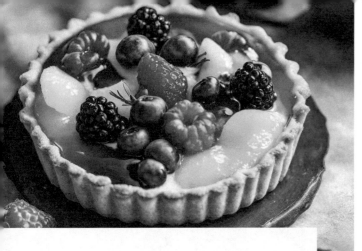

Fruit Tart

(France)

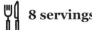 8 servings  30 minutes   20 minutes

INGREDIENTS

- 1 disc of ready-made or homemade shortcrust pastry
- 2 cups pastry cream
- 2 cups assorted fresh fruit (strawberries, kiwi, blueberries, etc.)
- 1/4 cup clear glaze for garnish

DIRECTIONS

Roll out the shortcrust pastry into a tart pan, prick the bottom with a fork, and bake blind at 350°F (175°C) until golden, about 20 minutes. Allow to cool, then fill with pastry cream and arrange the sliced fresh fruit on top. Heat the glaze until liquid and brush gently over the fruit to give it a shine. Chill in the refrigerator before serving.

CALORIES 320 KCAL	PROTEIN 5G	FATS 15G	FIBRE 2G

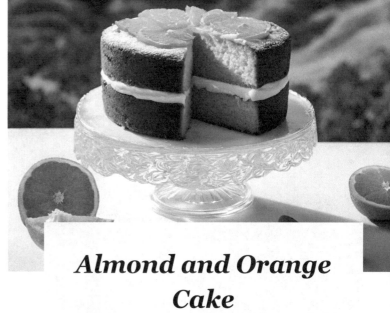

Almond and Orange Cake

(Spain, Andalusia)

 8 servings 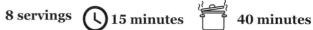 15 minutes   40 minutes

INGREDIENTS

- 2 cups ground almonds
- 1 cup granulated sugar
- 4 eggs
- Zest of 1 large orange
- Juice of 1 large orange
- 1 teaspoon baking powder
- Powdered sugar for dusting (optional)
- Sliced almonds for garnish (optional)

DIRECTIONS

Preheat your oven to 350°F (175°C), grease, and line an 8-inch round cake pan with parchment paper. In a large bowl, whisk eggs and sugar until fluffy, then stir in ground almonds, orange zest, juice, and baking powder until combined. Pour the batter into the pan, smooth the top, and bake for about 40 minutes or until a toothpick comes out clean. Allow to cool in the pan for 10 minutes, then transfer to a wire rack to cool completely. Dust with powdered sugar and garnish with sliced almonds before serving, if desired.

CALORIES 320 KCAL	PROTEIN 10G	FATS 18G	FIBRE 3G

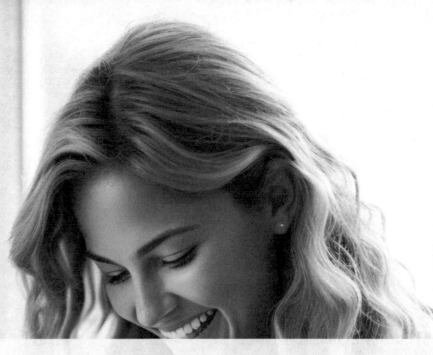

4-Weeks
Meal plan

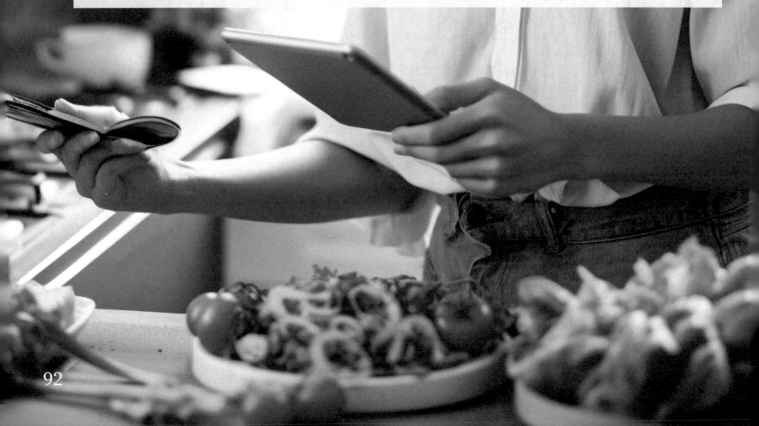

1 WEEK MEAL PLAN

	BREAKFAST	LUNCH	DINNER
MONDAY	Greek Yogurt with Honey and Nuts 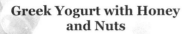	Red Lentil Soup 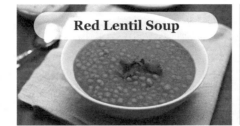	Seafood Paella 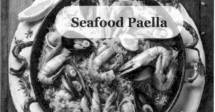
TUESDAY	Barley Porridge with Fresh Fruit	Chicken Tagine with Olives and Preserved Lemons 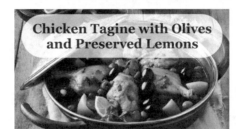	Lemon and Oregano Chicken 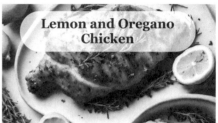
WEDNESDAY	Whole Wheat Crepes with Apricot Compote 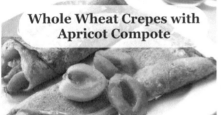	Mixed Fish Grill 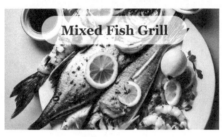	Farro with Cherry Tomatoes and Basil 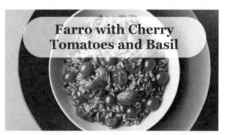
THURSDAY	Herb Omelette with Queso Fresco 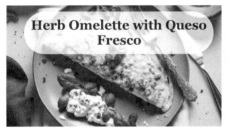	White Bean Cassoulet 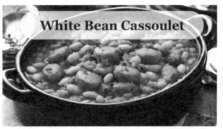	Fish Tagine 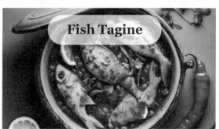
FRIDAY	Rye Bread with Avocado and Smoked Salmon 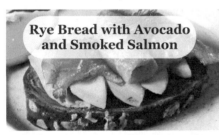	Moussaka 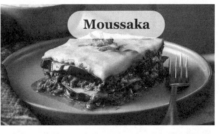	Farro with Artichokes and Pecorino 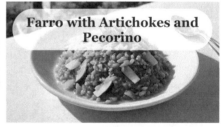
SATURDAY	Quinoa Salad with Citrus and Mint 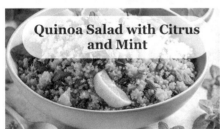	Baked Chicken with Potatoes and Rosemary 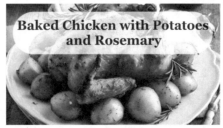	Whole Wheat Couscous with Vegetables 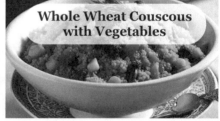
SUNDAY	Chickpea Flour Pancakes with Vegetables 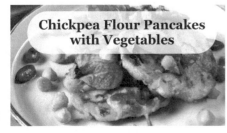	Squid Tagine 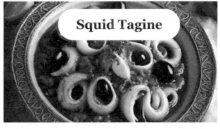	Whole Grain Polenta with Vegetable Ragù 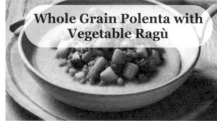

2 WEEK MEAL PLAN

	BREAKFAST	LUNCH	DINNER
MONDAY	Chilled Cucumber and Yogurt Gazpacho 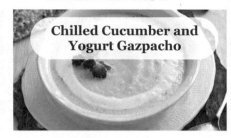	Chickpea and Spinach Soup 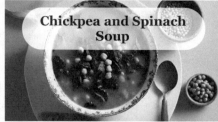	Grilled Lamb Chops 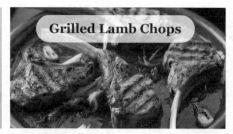
TUESDAY	Barley Porridge with Fresh Fruit 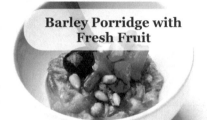	Fideuà 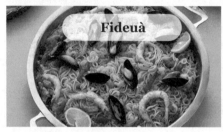	Fish Couscous 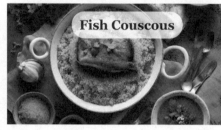
WEDNESDAY	Herb Omelette with Queso Fresco 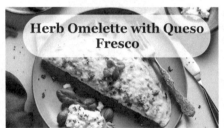	Farro with Artichokes and Pecorino 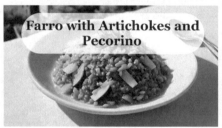	Paella Valenciana with Chicken and Rabbit 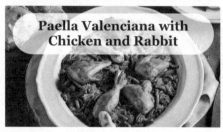
THURSDAY	Farro with Cherry Tomatoes and Basil 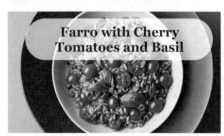	Soupe de Poisson 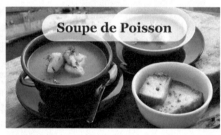	Chickpea and Vegetable Tagine 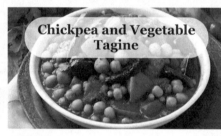
FRIDAY	Greek Yogurt with Honey and Nuts 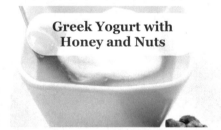	Acqua Pazza Fish 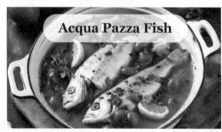	Lavraki Plaki 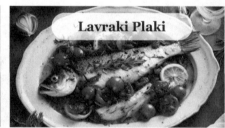
SATURDAY	Olives and Feta Cheese with Olive Oil 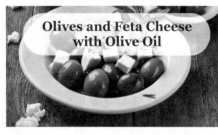	Paella Valenciana with Chicken and Rabbit 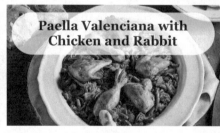	Grilled Whole Grain Polenta with Tomato Sauce 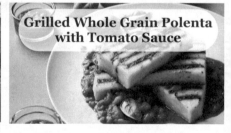
SUNDAY	Quinoa Salad with Citrus and Mint 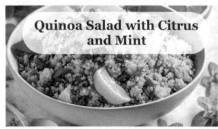	Bouillabaisse 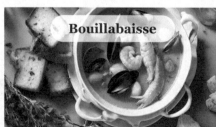	Moules Marinières 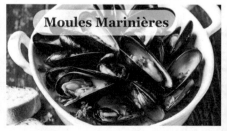

3 WEEK MEAL PLAN

	BREAKFAST	LUNCH	DINNER
MONDAY	Greek Yogurt with Honey and Nuts 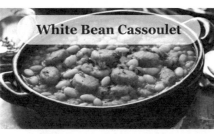	White Bean Cassoulet 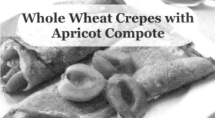	Chicken Fricassee 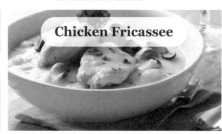
TUESDAY	Whole Wheat Crepes with Apricot Compote 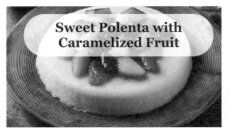	Falafel 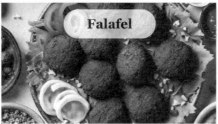	Caldeirada 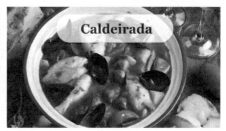
WEDNESDAY	Sweet Polenta with Caramelized Fruit 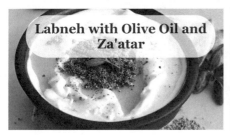	Fava Beans and Chicory 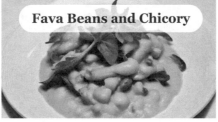	Chicken Provençal 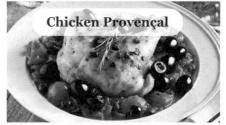
THURSDAY	Labneh with Olive Oil and Za'atar 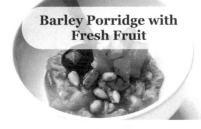	Moroccan Split Pea Soup 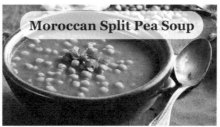	Şiş Tavuk 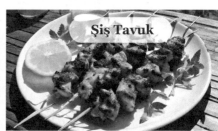
FRIDAY	Barley Porridge with Fresh Fruit 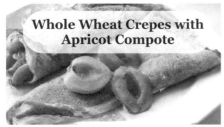	Bissara 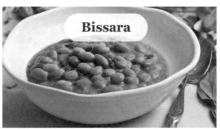	Oven-Roasted Pork Loin with Potatoes 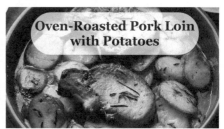
SATURDAY	Whole Wheat Crepes with Apricot Compote 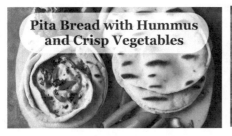	Loubia 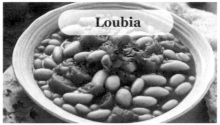	Octopus Salad 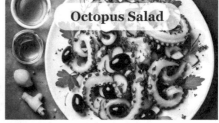
SUNDAY	Pita Bread with Hummus and Crisp Vegetables	Feijoada Transmontana 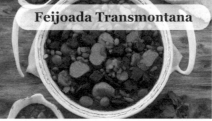	Whole Grain Mushroom Risotto 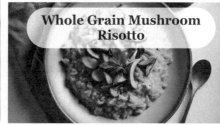

4 WEEK MEAL PLAN

	BREAKFAST	LUNCH	DINNER
MONDAY	Msemen with Honey and Almonds 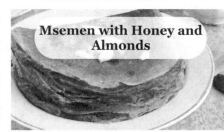	Provençal Quinoa Gratin 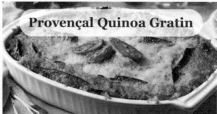	Grilled Lamb Chops 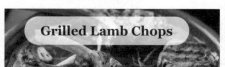
TUESDAY	Rye Bread with Avocado and Smoked Salmon 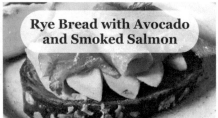	Fagioli all'Uccelletto 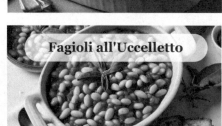	Chicken Milanese 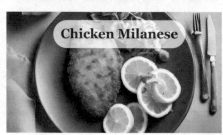
WEDNESDAY	Whole Wheat Crepes with Apricot Compote 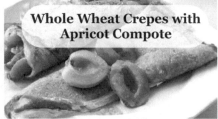	Red Lentil Soup 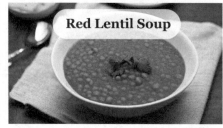	Mixed Fish Grill 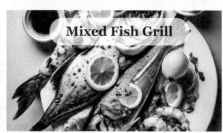
THURSDAY	Msemen with Honey and Almonds 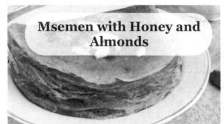	Moroccan Split Pea Soup 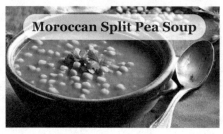	Chicken Shawarma 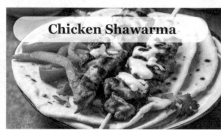
FRIDAY	Barley Porridge with Fresh Fruit 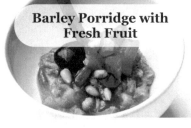	Acquacotta with Beans and Vegetables 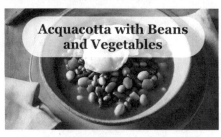	Şiş Tavuk 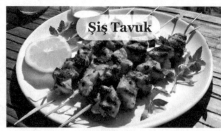
SATURDAY	Greek Yogurt with Honey and Nuts 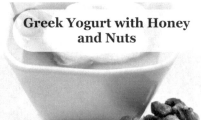	Chickpea and Spinach Soup 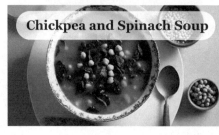	Fish Tagine 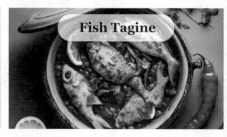
SUNDAY	Spinach and Ricotta Savory Pie 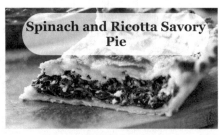	Chicken Provençal 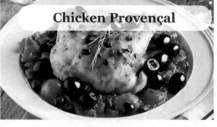	Bouillabaisse 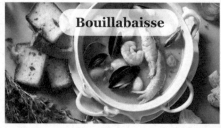

COOKING
CONVERSION
CHART

Measurement

CUP	ONCES	MILLILITERS	TABLESPOONS
8 cup	64 oz	1895 ml	128
6 cup	48 oz	1420 ml	96
5 cup	40 oz	1180 ml	80
4 cup	32 oz	960 ml	64
2 cup	16 oz	480 ml	32
1 cup	8 oz	240 ml	16
3/4 cup	6 oz	177 ml	12
2/3 cup	5 oz	158 ml	11
1/2 cup	4 oz	118 ml	8
3/8 cup	3 oz	90 ml	6
1/3 cup	2.5 oz	79 ml	5.5
1/4 cup	2 oz	59 ml	4
1/8 cup	1 oz	30 ml	3
1/16 cup	1/2 oz	15 ml	1

Temperature

FAHRENHEIT	CELSIUS
100 ºF	37 ºC
150 ºF	65 ºC
200 ºF	93 ºC
250 ºF	121 ºC
300 ºF	150 ºC
325 ºF	160 ºC
350 ºF	180 ºC
375 ºF	190 ºC
400 ºF	200 ºC
425 ºF	220 ºC
450 ºF	230 ºC
500 ºF	260 ºC
525 ºF	274 ºC
550 ºF	288 ºC

Weight

IMPERIAL	METRIC
1/2 oz	15 g
1 oz	29 g
2 oz	57 g
3 oz	85 g
4 oz	113 g
5 oz	141 g
6 oz	170 g
8 oz	227 g
10 oz	283 g
12 oz	340 g
13 oz	369 g
14 oz	397 g
15 oz	425 g
1 lb	453 g

SCAN THE QR CODE AND ACCESS YOUR BONUSES

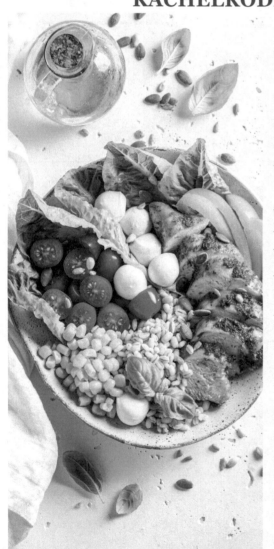

In conclusion, this journey through the Mediterranean diet has allowed us to uncover its nutritional richness and culinary delight and embrace a way of life that celebrates sharing, seasonality, and respect for nature. The recipes and stories shared within these pages invite reconnecting with the roots of one of the world's healthiest and most sustainable dietary traditions.

By incorporating the Mediterranean diet into our daily lives, we have the opportunity to improve our health and contribute to the health of our planet. It's a dietary choice that extends beyond mere eating, becoming an act of care for ourselves and the surrounding environment.

I hope the information, recipes, and tips provided in this book have inspired you to integrate the teachings of the Mediterranean diet into your life and discover the joy of mindful and joyous eating. May you find joy in every shared meal, health in every prepared dish, and beauty in the simplicity of the ingredients you choose.

I wish you a journey filled with culinary discoveries and satisfaction. I hope that the principles of the Mediterranean diet may enrich your table and your life for many years to come. Thank you for joining me on this culinary adventure. Safe travels into the world of the Mediterranean diet, where each bite is a step towards well-being.

Rachel Rodriguez

Made in United States
Troutdale, OR
11/13/2024

24798410R00055